T0142556

INSTRUCTION MANUAL IN OBSTETRICS

VOLUME ONE

INSTRUCTION MANUAL IN OBSTETRICS

DR. LAMIAA MOUSA AL-MADANY

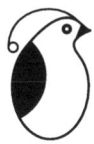

PARTRIDGE

Copyright © 2017 by Lamiaa Mousa AL-Madany.

Library of Congress Control Number: 2017953954
ISBN: Hardcover 978-1-5437-4252-7
Softcover 978-1-5437-4251-0
eBook 978-1-5437-4250-3

All rights reserved. No part of this book may be used or reproduced by any means, graphic, electronic, or mechanical, including photocopying, recording, taping or by any information storage retrieval system without the written permission of the author except in the case of brief quotations embodied in critical articles and reviews.

Because of the dynamic nature of the Internet, any web addresses or links contained in this book may have changed since publication and may no longer be valid. The views expressed in this work are solely those of the author and do not necessarily reflect the views of the publisher, and the publisher hereby disclaims any responsibility for them.

Print information available on the last page.

To order additional copies of this book, contact
Toll Free 800 101 2657 (Singapore)
Toll Free 1 800 81 7340 (Malaysia)
orders.singapore@partridgepublishing.com

www.partridgepublishing.com/singapore

7.2 Management of polyhydramnios 24
8 Intrauterine growth restriction 25
8.1 Management of IUGR 25
8.2 Asymmetrical IUGR 26
8.3 Management of Asymmetrical IUGR 27
9 Urinary tract infections in pregnancy 28
9.1 Type of Urinary tract infections 28
9.2 Management of Urinary tract infections 29
10 Intrahepatic cholestasis of pregnancy 30
10.1 Management of Intrahepatic cholestasis of pregnancy 30
10.2 Management of Intrahepatic cholestasis of pregnancy2 31
11 Varicella-zoster virus in pregnancy 32
11.1 VZV complication 33
11.2 VZV diagnosis 34
11.3 VZV Treatment 35
11.4 Management of VZV Exposure during pregnancy ... 36
12 Toxoplasmosis and pregnancy 38
12.1 Toxoplasma infection during pregnancy 38
12.2 Toxoplasma infection diagnosis 39
12.3 Tratment of Toxoplasma infection during pregnancy 40
13 Gonorrheal infection in pregnancy 41
14 Hepatitis B during pregnancy 42
14.1 Management of acute HBV 42
14.2 Chronic HBV 43
14.3 Breast-feeding in patient with HBV 44
15 Cytomegalovirus infection in pregnancy 45
15.1 Cytomegalovirus infection (CMV) 45
15.2 Maternal CMV infection 46
15.3 Prenatal diagnosis 47
16 Genital herpes simplex virus (HSV) infection 48
16.1 Genital herpes simplex virus (HSV) infection 48

Table of Contents

1 Follow up of normal pregnancy 1
2 First trimester vaginal bleeding 3
2.1 Management &treatment of first trimester vaginal bleeding 4
2.2 Vaginal bleeding with positive pregnancy test 5
2.3 Ultrasound with vaginal bleeding 6
2.4 Septic abortion 7
3 Venous thromboprophylactic 8
3.1 Risk assessment od venous thromboembolism in antenatal patient 9
3.2 Risk assessment od venous thromboembolism in postenatal patient 11
4 Thrombocytopenia during pregnancy 13
4.1 Management of patient with ITTP 14
4.2 Causes of Thrombocytopenia during pregnancy 15
5 Anemia in pregnancy 16
5.1 Definition of Anemia in pregnancy 16
5.2 Causes of anemia in pregnancy 17
5.3 Risk of sever anemia with pregnancy 17
5.4 Evaluation of pregnant patient with anemia 18
5.5 Investigate for macrocytic anemia 19
5.6 Treatment of anemia in pregnancy 20
6 Oligohydramnios 21
6.1 Causes of oligohydramnios 21
6.2 Management of oligohydramnios 22
7 Polyhydramnios 23
7.1 Causes of oligohydramnios 23

16.2 Genital Herpes during Labour or <34 weeks gestation 49
16.3 Genital Herpes at >34 weeks 50
17 Parvovirus B19 infection 51
17.1 Parvovirus B19 infection 51
17.2 Parvovirus B19 infection diagnosia 52
18 Syphilis in pregnancy 53
18.1 Stages of Syphilis during pregnancy 53
18.2 Syphilis complicating pregnancy 54
18.3 Syphilis Diagnosis 55
18.4 Management of syphilis in pregnancy 56
19 Sickle cell disease with pregnancy 57
19.1 Prepregnancy evaluation of sickle cell disease 57
19.2 Prepregnancy Management of medications & immunization in sickle cell disease patient 58
19.3 Risk of sickle cell disease on pregnancy 59
19.4 Prenatal care of sickle cell disease "HbSS, HbSC, HbS/beta-thal 60
19.5 Management of complication 61
20 Hypothyroidism 62
20.1 Hypothyroidism in preconception 62
20.2 Thyroid disease in pregnancy 63
21 Diabetes 64
21.1 Gestational diabetes 64
21.2 screen for gestational diabetis 65
21.3 Follow up of gestational diabetis 66
22 Preconception type 1&type 2 diabetes mellitus 67
22.1 Preconception management of type 1&type 2 diabetes mellitus 67
22.2 Preconception management of type 1&type 2 diabetes mellitus 68
22.3 ANC follow up for type 1&type 2 diabetes mellitus 69
22.4 Intrapartum care for patient with diabetis mellitus 70

22.5 Post natal care with diabetis mellitus type1&2 71
23 Hypertension in pregnancy 72
23.1 Risk factors for pre-eclampsia 73
23.2 HTN disease in pregnancy 73
23.3 Chronic hypertension in pregnancy 74
23.4 Antihypertensive drug during pregnancy..... 76
23.5 BP target in treatment of HTN disease in pregnancy 77
23.6 Time of delivery in chronic HTN patient 77
23.7 Post partum follow up with chronic HTN 78
23.8 Gestational hypertension classification..... 79
23.9 Gestational hypertension 80
23.10 Management of pregnancy with gestational HTN 80
23.11 Preconception advice 81
23.12 ANC follow up of patient with gestational hypertension 82
23.13 Time of delivery 83
23.14 Postnatal investigation, monitoring and treatment..... 84
24 Protein S deficiency..... 85
24.1 Management of protein S deficiency 86
25 Systemic lupus erythematosus..... 87
25.1 Clinical course of SLE in pregnancy..... 87
25.2 The exacerbation of renal disease in SLE patient.... 88
25.3 Pregnancy following renal transplantation..... 89
25.4 Treatment of patient with SLE Recommendation..... 89
25.5 ANC follow up for patient with SLE 90
25.6 Monitoring of SLE patient in the last trimester 90
25.7 Management of patient with SLE in the postpartum period..... 91
25.8 Drug safe for the nursing infant..... 91
25.9 Treatment of active disease. 92
25.10 Drug with Moderate to high risk of fetal harm..... 92
25.11 Drug with Minimal fetal and maternal risk..... 93

25.12 Drug with Selective use allowed during pregnancy 94
25.13 Thrombocytopenia in SLE 95
26 Pregnancy with kidney disease 96
26.1 Preconception advice for effect of pregnancy on kidney disease 96
26.2 Effect of pregnancy on renal function RF 97
26.3 Management of pregnant women with renal disease 98
26.4 Special situation in pregnancy with renal disease 99
27 Rh and other blood group alloimmunizations 101
27.1 Follow up of Rh-negative blood group 101
27.2 ANC follow up and Monitored for the development of fetal anemia 102
27.3 Management of subsequent Alloimmune pregnancy 103
28. Epilepsy in pregnancy 104
28.1 Preconception advice 104
28.2 Management of epileptic patient during pregnancy 105
28.3 Mode of delivery in patient with epilepsy 106
28.4 Post partum care for patient with epilepsy 106
29 Cardiac disease in pregnancy 107
29.1 type of cardiac diseas in pregnancy 107
29.2 Condition associated with maternal and fetal risk 108
29.3 ANC for patient with cardiac disease 109
29.4 Mode of delivery in cardiac patient 110
30 Diagnoses and Management of patient in Labor 113
30.1 Patient assessment in emergency room 114
30.2 Patient assessment in labor room 115
30.3 Third Stage of Labor 116
30.4 Category of the CTG 117
30.5 Categorization of Fetal Heart Rate 118
30.6 Management of CTG: 120

30.7 Classification of Fetal Blood Sample Results 124
31 Regimen for Syntocinon Infusion..... 125
32 Cord Blood Sampling 129
33 Guidelines for the care of women' presenting in labor.... 130
34 Group B Streptococcus (GBS) in Labor 131
34.1 Prevention of Perinatal Group B Streptococcal (GBS) Disease 131
34.2 Recommended regimens for intrapartum antibiotic prophylaxis for prevention of early-onset group B streptococcal (GBS) disease 132
34.3 Group B Streptococcus(GBS) in Labor Pathway... 133
35 Induction of Labor (IOL) 134
35.1 Defention needed in induction of labor..... 135
35.2 Modified Bishop Scoring System..... 136
35.3 Ripening / induction: of unfavorable Cervix..... 137
35.4 Induction With a Favorable Cervix..... 138
35.5 Induction of labor pathway 139
36 The Management of Third- and Fourth-Degree Perineal Tears 140
36.1 Repair of third- and fourth-degree pathway..... 141
37 Labor Management of women with previous Caesarean Section in..... 142
37.1 Planned vaginal birth after ceaserian section..... 142
37.2 Labor &birth in previous Ceaserian section..... 143
37.3 Induction of labor in VBAC pathway1 144
37.4 Unfavorable cervix 145
37.5 Favorable cervix..... 146
37.6 Induction of labor in previous scar pathway2..... 147
38 Spontaneous Ruptures OF Membranes (SROM)..... 148
38.1 Diagnosis 148
38.2 Management of SROM>37wks 149
38.3 Spontaneous rupture of membrane (PPROM)<37wks pathway 150

39 PRE-TERMLABOUR 151
39.1 Defention of preterm labour 151
39.2 Initial assessment 151
39.3 Pre term labor guidline 152
40 Corticosteroids 153
40.1 Indication for administration of corticosteroids 153
40.2 Administration of corticosteroid in special situation 154
40.3 Type, dose administration corticosteroids 155
41 Tocolytics 156
41.1 Atosiban 157
42 Hypertensive disease in pregnancy 158
42.1 Definitions of HTN disease in pregnancy 158
42.2 Preeclampsia definition 159
42.3 Preeclampsia management pathway 160
42.4 Features of Severe preeclampsia 161
43 Eclampsia 162
43.1 Eclampsia management pathway 162
43.2 Recurrence of seizures management pathway 163
43.3 Post Partum Fluid Protocol – Pre Eclampsia 165
43.4 Anti hypertensive 166
43.5 Choice of antihypertensive 166
43.6 2nd line of antihypertensive agent pathway 167
43.7 Seizure prophylaxis Magnesium sulphate protocol 168
43.8 Treatment Of Magnesium Toxicity 169
44 Management of Laboring Women with IDDM/ Gestational Diabetes 170
44.1 Time of delivery 170
44.2 Methods of delivery 171
44.3 Control of blood glucose during latent phase of labor 171
44.4 Control of blood glucose during during active phase &NPO for elective ceaserian section 172

44.5 Diabetic patient Post delivery pathway 173
44.6 Diabetic patient on insulin with preterm labor 174
44.7 Diabetic pregnant women with KDA..... 175
44.8 Management of DKA 175
45 Antepartum Hemorrhage 176
45.1 Classification of the severity of APH. 176
45.2 Causes Antepartum haemorrhage..... 177
45.3 Complications of APH..... 178
45.4 The main therapeutic goal of management of massive blood loss:..... 179
45.5 Fluid therapy and blood product transfusion..... 180
45.6 Antepartum Hemorrhage pathway 181
46 Genital Herpes during pregnancy 182
46.1 Protocol for Genital Herpes during Labour or <34 weeks gestation 182
46.2 Protocol for Genital Herpes during Labour or >34 weeks gestation..... 183
47 Instrumental delivery pre-requisites 184
47.1 Pre-requisites for instrumental vaginal delivery 184
47.2 Instrumental delivery application pathway..... 185
48 Pre Requisites for Caesarean Section guideline 186
49 Caesarean Section..... 187
49.1 Classification Of Caesarean Sections..... 187
49.2 second Stage Caesarean Section pathway 188
49.3 Prophylactic Antibiotics..... 189
50 Breech Delivery 190
50.1 Management of Breech Presentation in laboring pathway (Expected and Unexpected Breech) 191
50.2 Complecated breech delivery pathway 193
51 Twin Delivery 194
51.1 Twin management pathway 194
51.2 Twin delivery Management pathway 195
51.3 Analgesia 196
52 Shoulder Dystocia management pathway 197

53 Management of Cord Prolapse 198
53.1 Definitions Cord Presentation 198
53.2 Cord prolapse management pathway 199
54 Uterine Inversion 200
54.1 Suspect uterine inversion 200
54.2 Management of uterine inversion 201
55 Ruptured uterus 202
55.1 Risk factors for uterine rupture 202
55.2 Ruptured uterus management pathway 203
56 Retained Placenta 204
56.1 Definition 204
56.2 Retained placenta management 204
57 Care plan for women in labor if blood not available 205
57.1 Management Of Postpartum Anaemia 205
57.2 Management in active hemorrhage in labor if blood not avialable 206
57.3 1st step in active hemorrhage management 206
57.4 2nd step in active hemorrhage management pathway 207
57.5 Surgical management of post partum hemorrhage pathway 208
58 Management of Post Partum Hemorrhage 209
58.1 Risk Factors for Post Partum Hemorrhage 209
58.2 Definition& general measure to stabilize patient with PPH pathway 210
59 Massive transfusion 211
59.1 Management of patient with massive blood loss 211
59.2 Treatment of patient with severe hypovolemia or hypovolemic shock 212
59.3 Complication of massive blood transfusion 213
59.4 If the Patient require blood transfusion>5 unit 214
59.5 Complication of massive blood transfusion 215
59.6 Causes for PPH 'the four Ts' 218
59.7 Medical Management of uterine atony pathway 219
59.8 Surgical management of uterine atony pathway 220

60 Intra-Partum Collapse 221
60.1 Uterine Rupture 221
60.2 Eclampsia 221
60.3 Pulmonary Embolism Amniotic Fluid Embolism 222
60.4 Neurological Causes 223
60.5 Cardiac causes. 223
60.6 Cardiac Arrest 224
61 Management of delivery in cardiac disease patient 225
61.1 Aim and purpose 225
61.2 Timing of delivery 226
61.3 Mode of delivery 227
61.4 Prophylaxis antibiotics in cardiac patient 228
61.5 Post-partum period in cardiac patient 229
62 Extremely Premature Babies between22and26weeks Gestation 230
62.1 Action in Established Pre-term Labour pathway 230
63 Late inter-uterine death and still birth 231
63.1 Definition 231
63.2 Diagnosis 231
63.3 Communication 232
63.4 Isoimmunisation prevention 232
63.5 Mode of delivery and timing 233
63.6 Mode of delivery 234
63.7 IOL see flowchart 235
63.8 Investigations 237
64 Obstetric temple 238
64.1 Temple of vacuum delivery 238
64.2 Temple of forceps delivery 238
64.3 Temple of shoulder dystocia 238
65 Reference 243
65.1 chapter 1 reference 243
65.2 chapter 2 reference 243
65.3 chapter 3 referance 244
65.4 Chapter 4 reference 245
65.5 Chapter 5 Reference 245

65.6 Chapter 6 Reference.....245
65.7 chapter 7 Reference 246
65.8 Chapter 8 Reference.....247
65.9 Chapter 9 Reference.....247
65.10 Chapter 10.....248
65.11 Chapter 11 Reference.....248
65.12 Chapter 12 Reference 249
65.13 Chapter 13 Reference 250
65.14 Chapter 14 Reference 250
65.15 Chapter 15 Reference: 251
65.16 Chapter 16 Reference 251
65.17 Chapter 17 reference.....251
65.18 Chapter 18 Referance 252
65.19 Chapter 19 Reference 252
65.20 Chapter 20 Reference.....253
65.21 Chapter 21 Reference.....254
65.22 Chapter 22 Reference 255
65.23 Chapter 23 Reference.....255
65.24 Chapter 25 Reference.....256
65.25 Chapter 26 reference.....257
65.26 Chapter 27 Reference.....257
65.27 Chapter 28 Reference.....258
65.28 Chapter 29 Reference.....259
65.29 Reference Section II Instruction manual in Labour room.....259

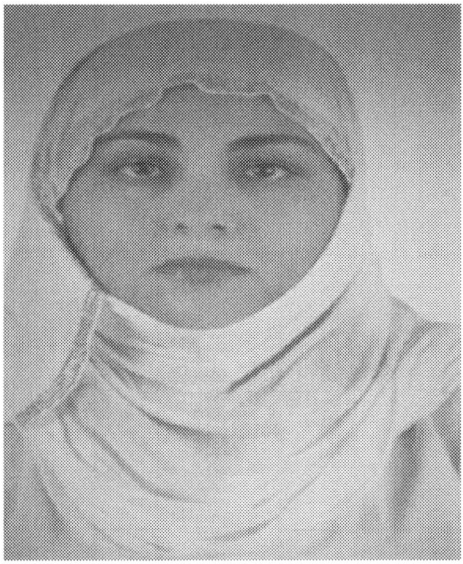

Dr: Lamiaa Mousa AL-Madany

Consultant Obstetric and Gynecology
Arab Board in Obstetric and Gynecology
MSC Quality & Safety in Healthcare Management
Certified Professional in Health & Hospital Administration
Member in Saudi Obstetric & Gynecological Society
Member of the European Society Of
Contraception And Reproductive Health
Member in Egyption Society of Maternal Fetal Medicine
Member in Saudi Osteoporosis Society
Member in Saudi Cancer Foundation

Instruction Manual in Obstetrics

Why to read this book

Evidence base knowledge is the most important factor to develop up to date standard of practice.

The aim of this book is to summarize the practical knowledge needed by an obstetrician and gynecologist to manage the patient in an out-patient clinic and labour room.

The information in this book is kept as headline which the physician will read, this information will not cover all the topic it will be the most important headline which is summarized in flow charts.

The aim of the flow chart is to carry out the short way which activate the physician's brain to remember by creating a brain map image.

Who is this book for?

If you can answer, "yes" to any of these:

1. Are you physician treating a female in obstetric and gynecology clinic?
2. Do you want to learn, understand, remember, and apply important updated evidence base information so you can treat your patient with high level of trust?
3. Do you want to pass the board exam, and learn to be a better obstetrician and gynecologist?

4. Do you prefer stimulating attractive challenging way of learning?

Then this book is for you.

After finishing this book you will be able to

1. Earn more self-confidence
2. Manage your patient in better way
3. earn your peer respect
4. stand in solid ground standing for medico legal cases
5. Strong base in teaching your junior
6. Gain more confidants to inter the board examination

Section I Instruction manual in Obstetric Clinic

1 Follow up of normal pregnancy

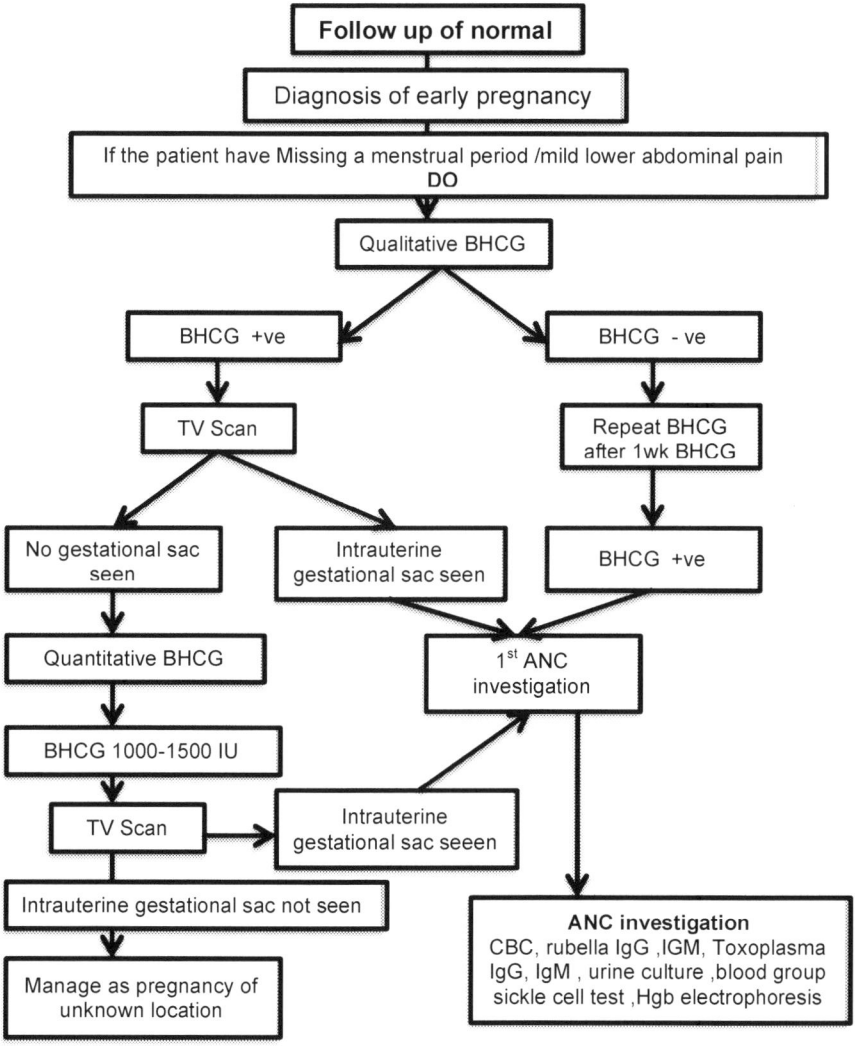

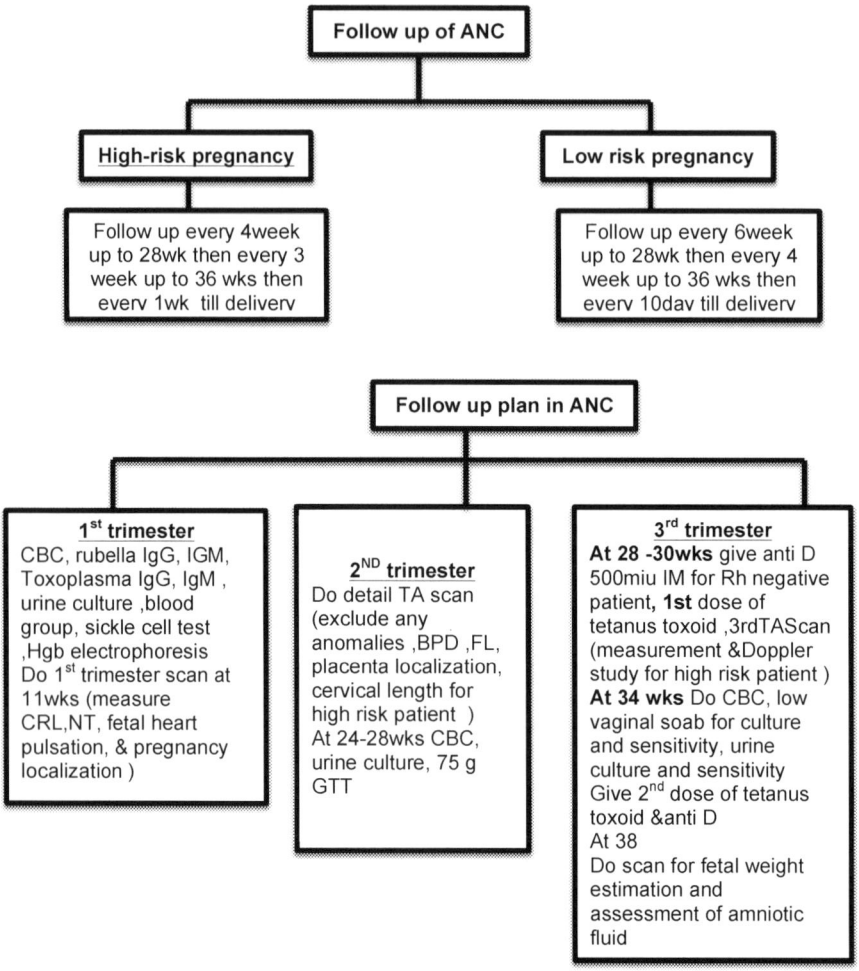
Follow up of ANC
High-risk pregnancy
Low risk pregnancy
Follow up every 4week up to 28wk then every 3 week up to 36 wks then every 1wk till delivery
Follow up every 6week up to 28wk then every 4 week up to 36 wks then every 10day till delivery
Follow up plan in ANC
1st trimester
CBC, rubella IgG, IGM, Toxoplasma IgG, IgM , urine culture ,blood group, sickle cell test ,Hgb electrophoresis
Do 1st trimester scan at 11wks (measure CRL,NT, fetal heart pulsation, & pregnancy localization)
2ND trimester
Do detail TA scan (exclude any anomalies ,BPD ,FL, placenta localization, cervical length for high risk patient)
At 24-28wks CBC, urine culture, 75 g GTT
3rd trimester
At 28 -30wks give anti D 500miu IM for Rh negative patient, 1st dose of tetanus toxoid ,3rdTAScan (measurement &Doppler study for high risk patient)
At 34 wks Do CBC, low vaginal soab for culture and sensitivity, urine culture and sensitivity
Give 2nd dose of tetanus toxoid &anti D
At 38
Do scan for fetal weight estimation and assessment of amniotic fluid

2 First trimester vaginal bleeding

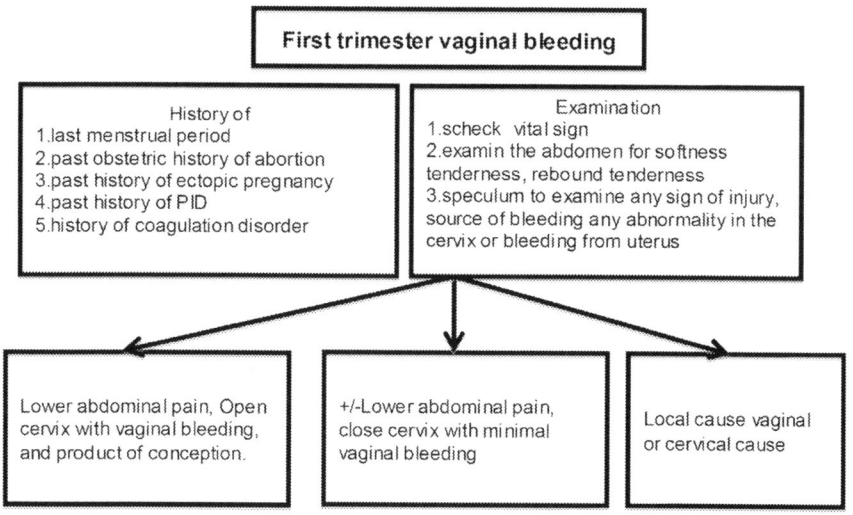

2.1 Management &treatment of first trimester vaginal bleeding

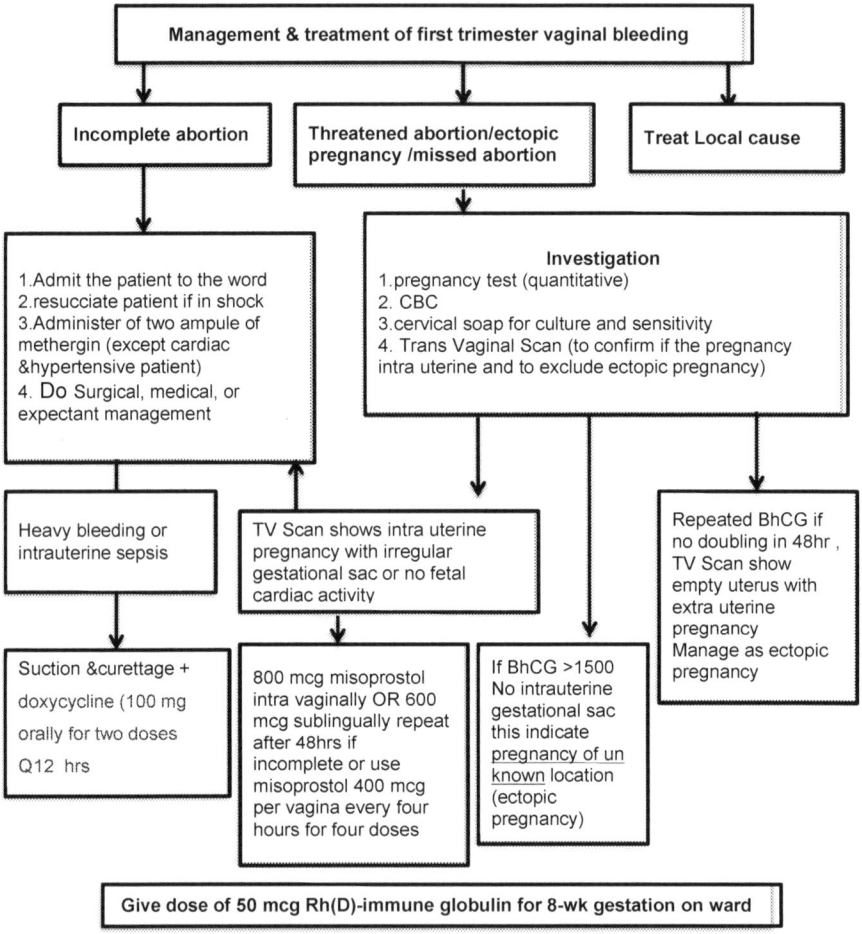

2.2 Vaginal bleeding with positive pregnancy test

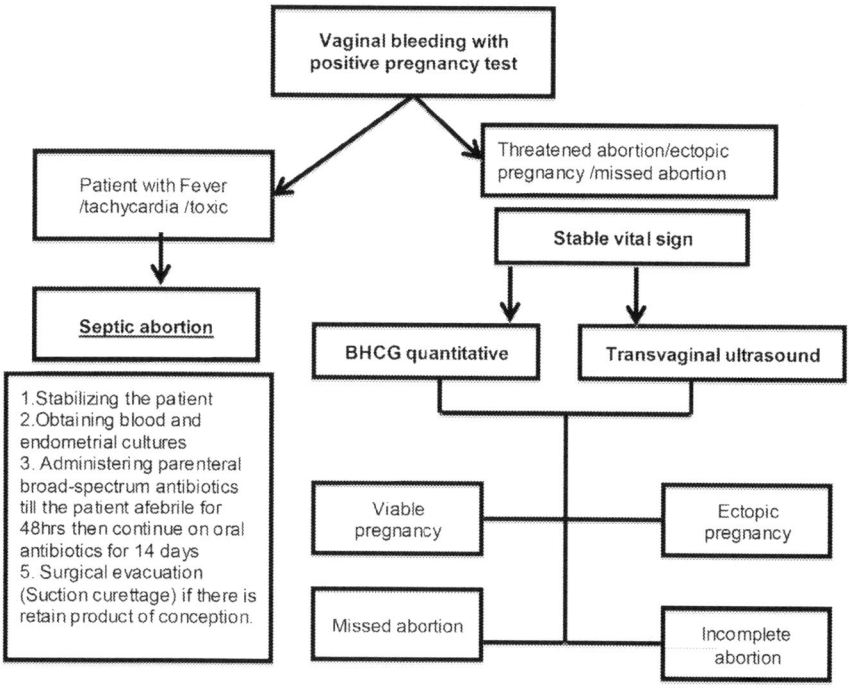

2.3 Ultrasound with vaginal bleeding

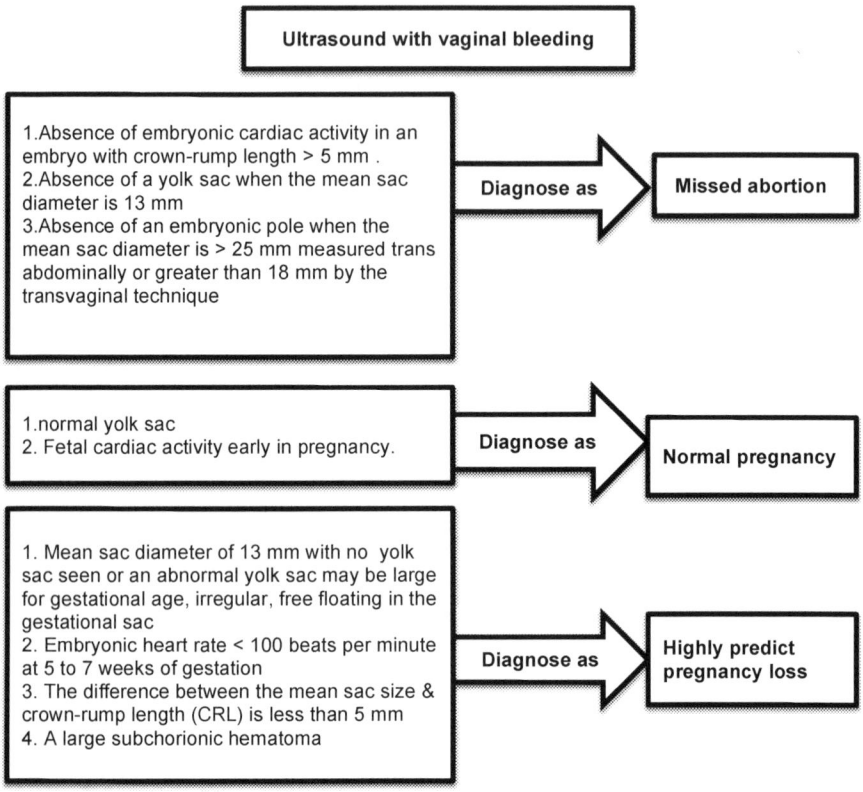

2.4 Septic abortion

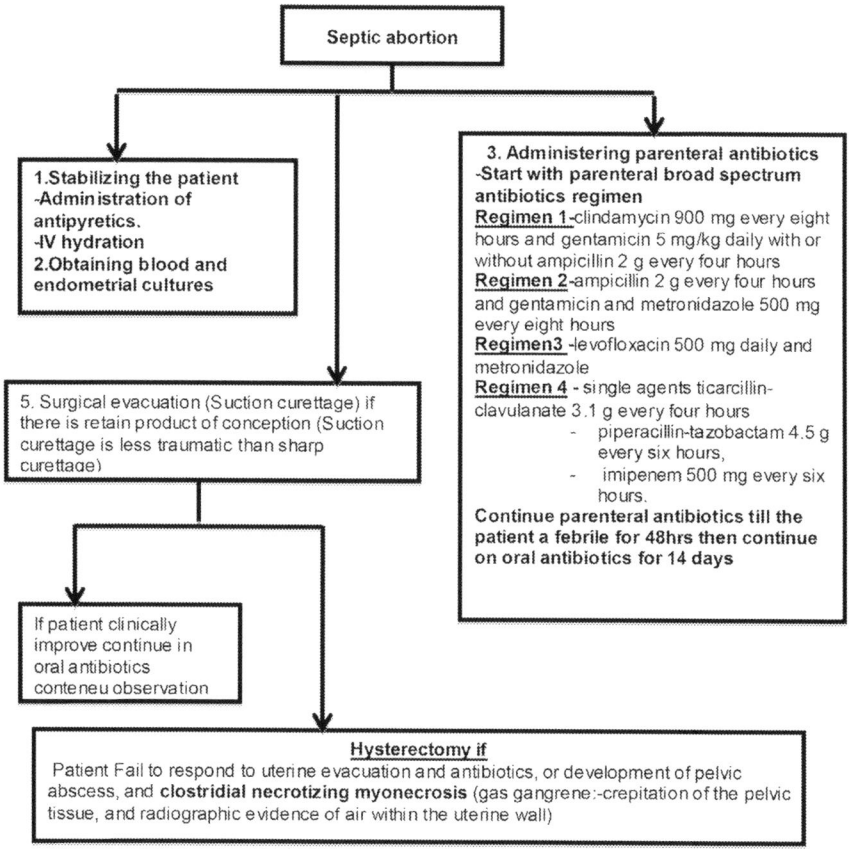

3 Venous thromboprophylactic

All women should undergo a documented of risk factors for VTE in early pregnancy or pre-pregnancy. Risk assessment should be repeated if the woman is ***admitted to hospital*** *for any reason or develops other intercurrent problems. Risk assessment should be repeated again* ***intrapartum*** *or* ***immediately postpartum.***

3.1 Risk assessment od venous thromboembolism in antenatal patient

High Risk Factor will score 4

1.Any previous VTE except a single event related to major surgery.
2.Pregnant women with APS.
3.Pregnant women with prior VTE
4.Pregnant women with prior arterial thrombosis.
5.Pregnant women with previous VTE associated with antithrombin deficiency.

Mild Risk Factor will score 1:

1.Obesity (BMI > 30 kg / m2.
2.Age > 35
3.Parity ≥ 3.
4.Smoker.
5.Gross varicose veins.
6.Current pre-eclampsia.
7.Immobility, e.g. paraplegia, PGP.
8.Family history of unprovoked or estrogen-
9.provoked VTE in first degree relative.
10.Family history of unprovoked or estrogen-
11.provoked VTE in first degree relative.
12.Low-risk thromphobophilia.
13Multiple pregnancies IVF/ART.

Intermediate Risk Factor will Score 3:

1.Hospital admission.
2.Single previous VTE related to major surgery.
3.High Risk thrombophilia + NO VTE.
4.Homozygous factor V Leiden.
5.Compound hetrozygote protein C deficiency.
6.Compound hetrozygote protein S deficiency.

Medical Comorbidities:

1.Patient with cancer.
2.Patient with heart failure.
3.Patient with IBD.
4.Patient with active SLE.
5.Patient with inflammatory polyarthropathy.
6.Patient with nephrotic syndrome.
7.Patient with Type I DM with nephropathy.
8.Patient with sickle cell disease, current IVDU.
9.Patient with current IVDU.
10.Patient with any surgical procedure e.g. appendectomy.

Transient Risk Factors: will receive LMWH as long the transient risk factor excess:

1.Patient with dehydration hyperemesis.
2.Patient with ovarian hyper stimulation syndrome.

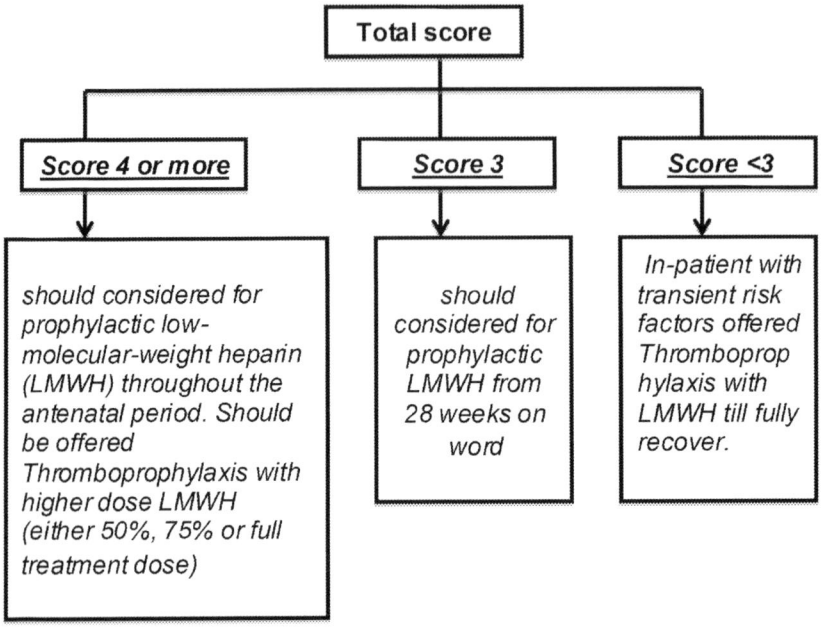

ANTENATAL PROPHYLACTIC DOSE OF LMWH:
Weight < 50 kg, give 20 mg enoxaparin daily.
Weight > 50-90 kg, give 40 mg enoxaparin daily.
Weight 91-130 kg, give 60 mg enoxaparin daily.
Weight 131-70 kg, give 80 mg enoxaparin daily.
Weight > 170 kg, give 6 mg /kg/day enoxaparin daily.

3.2 Risk assessment od venous thromboembolism in postenatal patient

High Risk Factor will score 4

1.Any previous VTE except a single event related to major surgery.
2.Patient with anyone requiring Antenatal LMWH
3.Patient with high risk thrombophilia homozygous factor V Leiden.
4.Patient with compound hetrozygote protein C or S deficiency.
5.Low Risk thrombophilia + family history of thromboembolic events.

Mild Risk Factor will score 1:

1.Obesity (BMI > 30 kg / m2.
2.Age > 35
3.Parity ≥ 3.
4.Patient with Elective Cesarean Section.
5.Gross varicose veins.
6.Current pre-eclampsia.
7.Immobility, e.g. paraplegia, PGP.
8.Family history of unprovoked or estrogen-9.provoked VTE in first-degree relative.
10.Low-risk thromphobophilia.
11.Patient with long distance travel.
12.Patient with multiple pregnancies.
13.Patient with pre-term delivery, in this pregnancy (<37+0 weeks).
14.Patient with stillbirth in this pregnancy.
15.Patient with Mid-cavity rotational or operative delivery.
16.Multiple pregnancies IVF/ART.
17.Patient with prolonged labour (> 24 hours).
18.Patient with PPH > 1 liter or blood transfusion.

Intermediate Risk Factor will Score 3:

1. Cesarean Section in labour.
2.BMI ≥ 40 kg / m2.
3.Readmission or prolonged admission (≥ 3 days) in the puerperium.
4.Any surgical procedure in the puerperium except immediate repair of the perineum.
5.Medical Comorbidities:
6.Patient with cancer.
7.Patient with heart failure.
8.Patient with IBD.
9.Patient with active SLE
10.Patient with inflammatory polyarthropathy.
11.Patient with nephrotic syndrome.
12.Patient with Type I DM with nephropathy
13.Patient with sickle cell disease, current IVDU 14.Patient with current IVDU.
15Patient with any surgical procedure e.g. appendectomy.

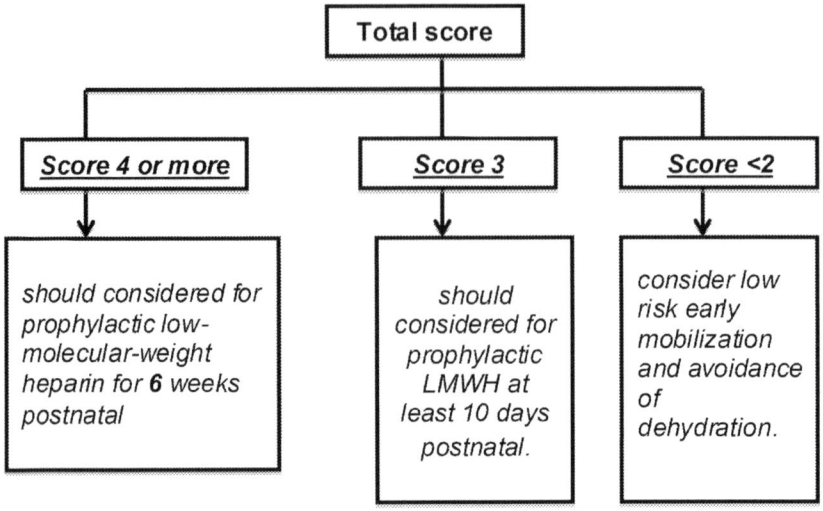

ANTENATAL PROPHYLACTIC DOSE OF LMWH:
Weight < 50 kg, give 20 mg enoxaparin daily.
Weight > 50-90 kg, give 40 mg enoxaparin daily.
Weight 91-130 kg, give 60 mg enoxaparin daily.
Weight 131-70 kg, give 80 mg enoxaparin daily.
Weight > 170 kg, give 6 mg /kg/day enoxaparin daily.

4 Thrombocytopenia during pregnancy

Thrombocytopenia during pregnancy

Thrombo-cytopenia during pregnancy

- **1.Gestational thrombocytopenia**
- **2.TTP/HUS**
- **3.Drug-induced ITTP**
- **4.Antiphospholipid syndrome thrombocytopenia**
- **4.ITTP Immune thrombocytopenic purpura**

Antenatal

- Forceps and vacuum assisted delivery are relatively contraindicated, if it is indicated use forceps rather than vacuum assisted deliver
-Cesarean delivery reserved only for standard obstetrical indications

Post natal

Antiplatelet drugs (eg, aspirin, nonsteroidal antiinflammatory drugs) should be avoided postpartum in women with thrombocytopenia.

4.1 Management of patient with ITTP

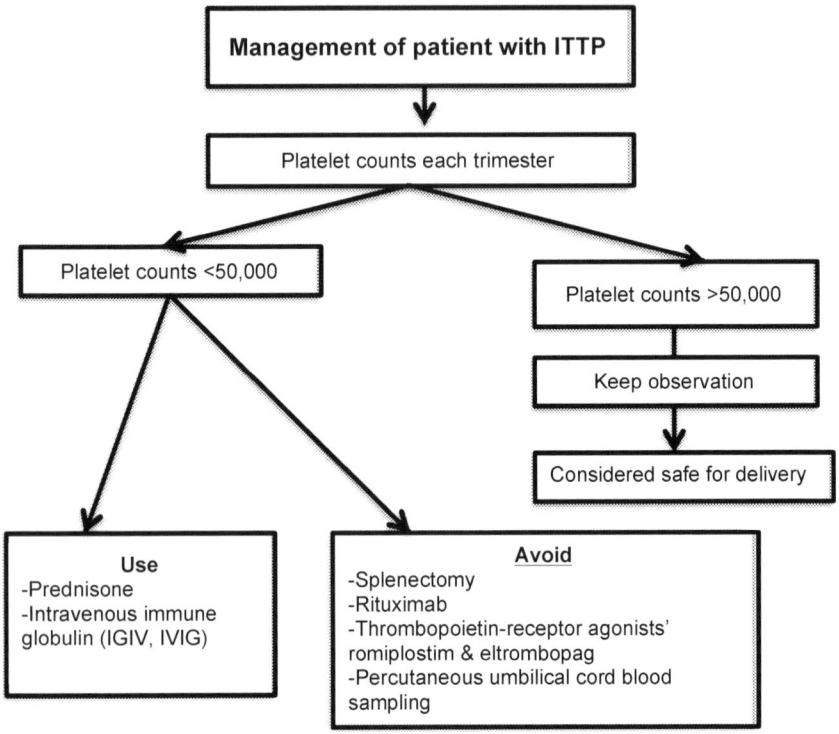

4.2 Causes of Thrombocytopenia during pregnancy

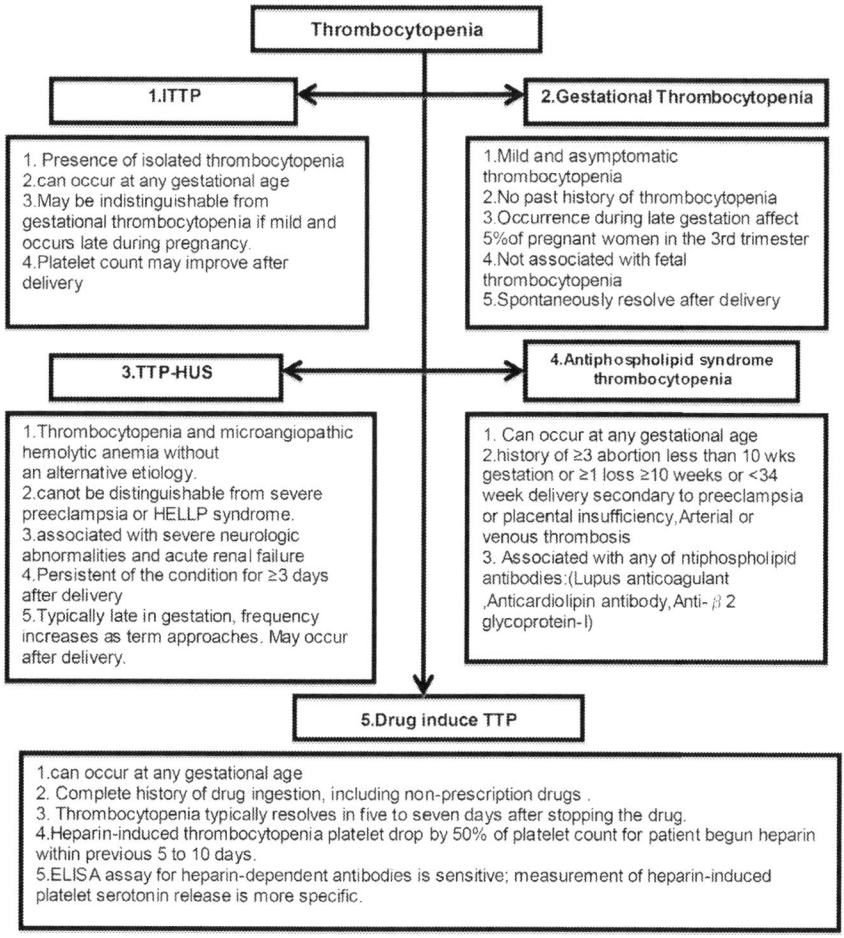

5 Anemia in pregnancy

5.1 Definition of Anemia in pregnancy

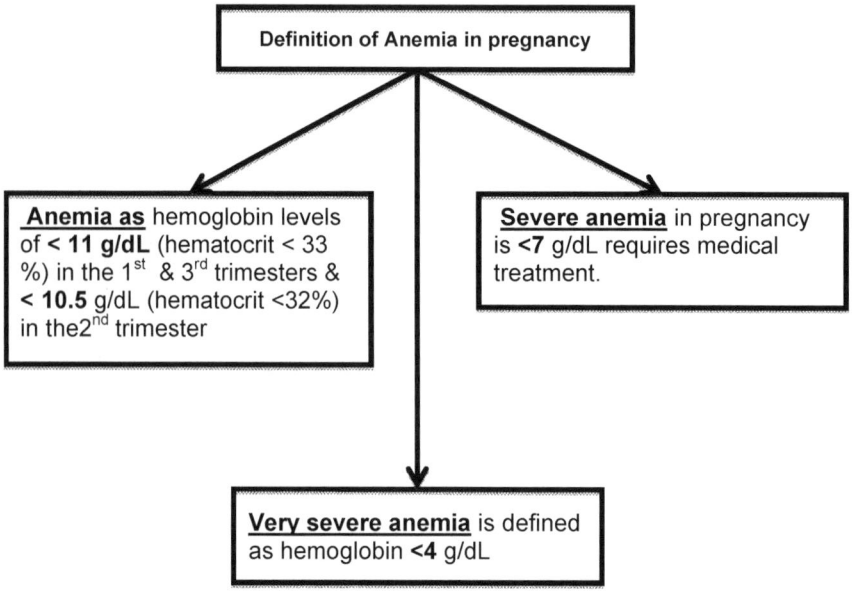

5.2 Causes of anemia in pregnancy

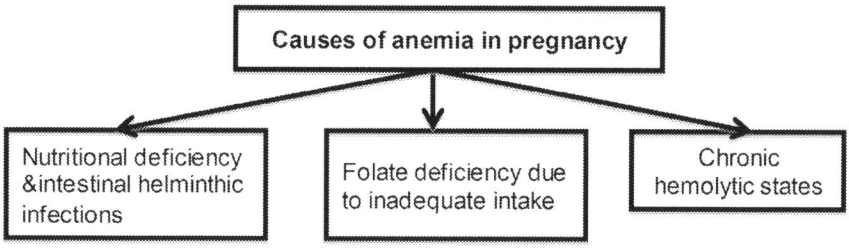

5.3 Risk of sever anemia with pregnancy

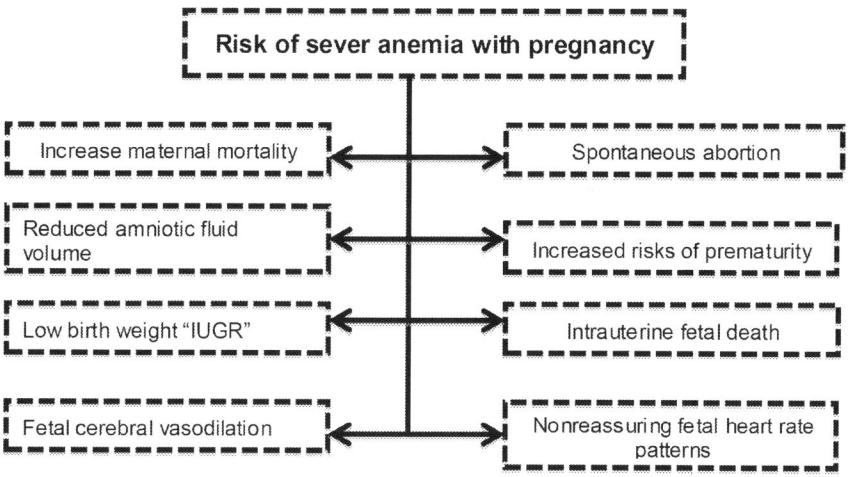

5.4 Evaluation of pregnant patient with anemia

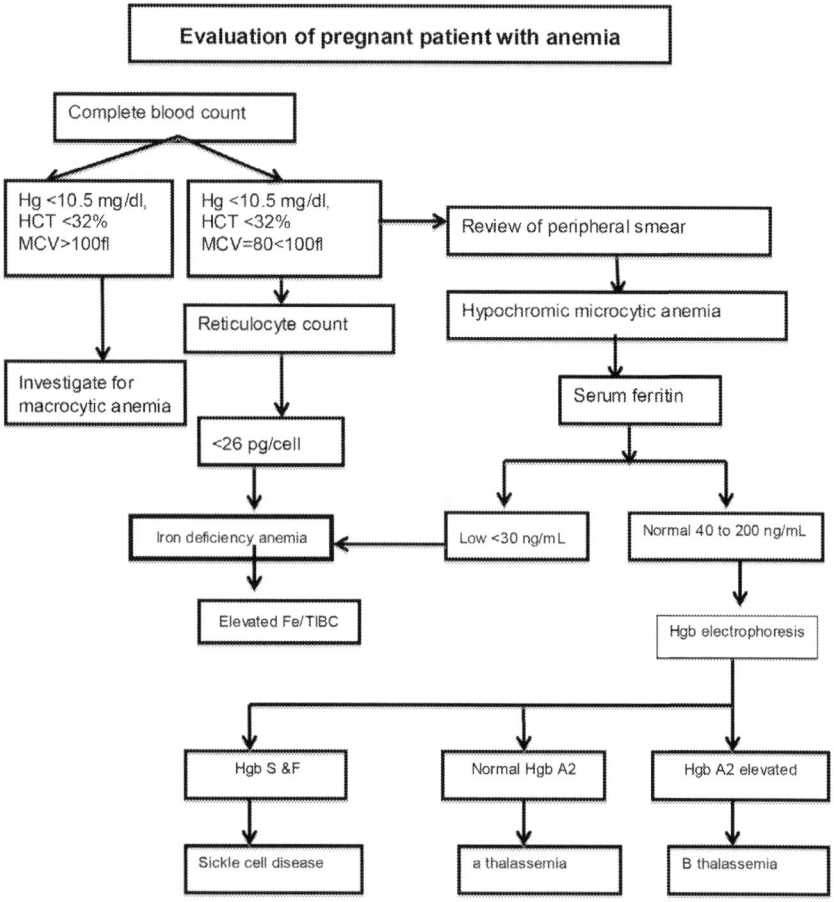

5.5 Investigate for macrocytic anemia

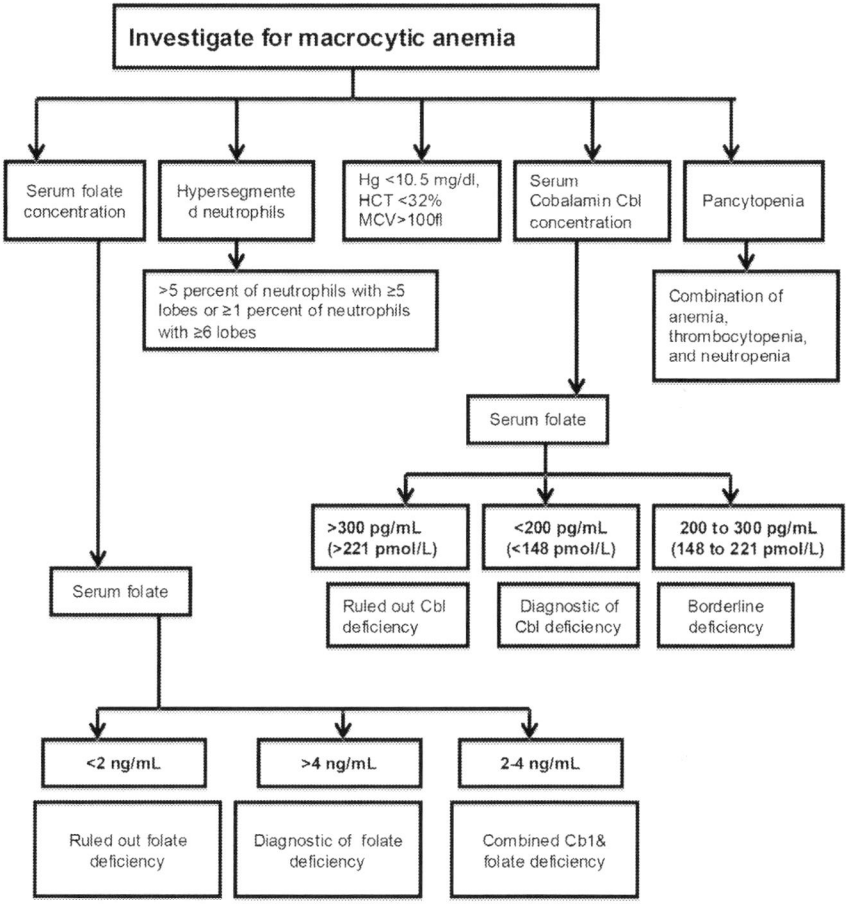

5.6 Treatment of anemia in pregnancy

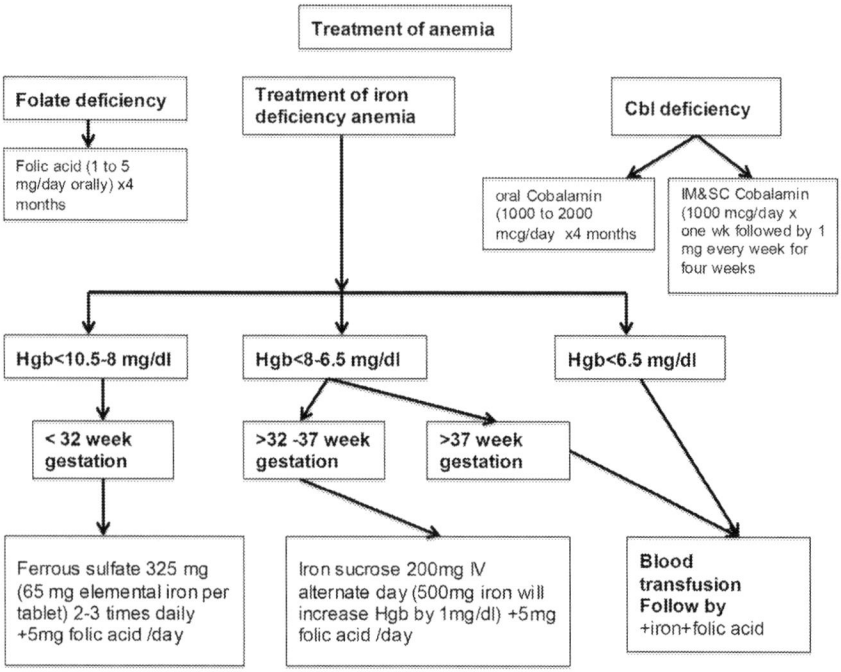

6 Oligohydramnios

6.1 Causes of oligohydramnios

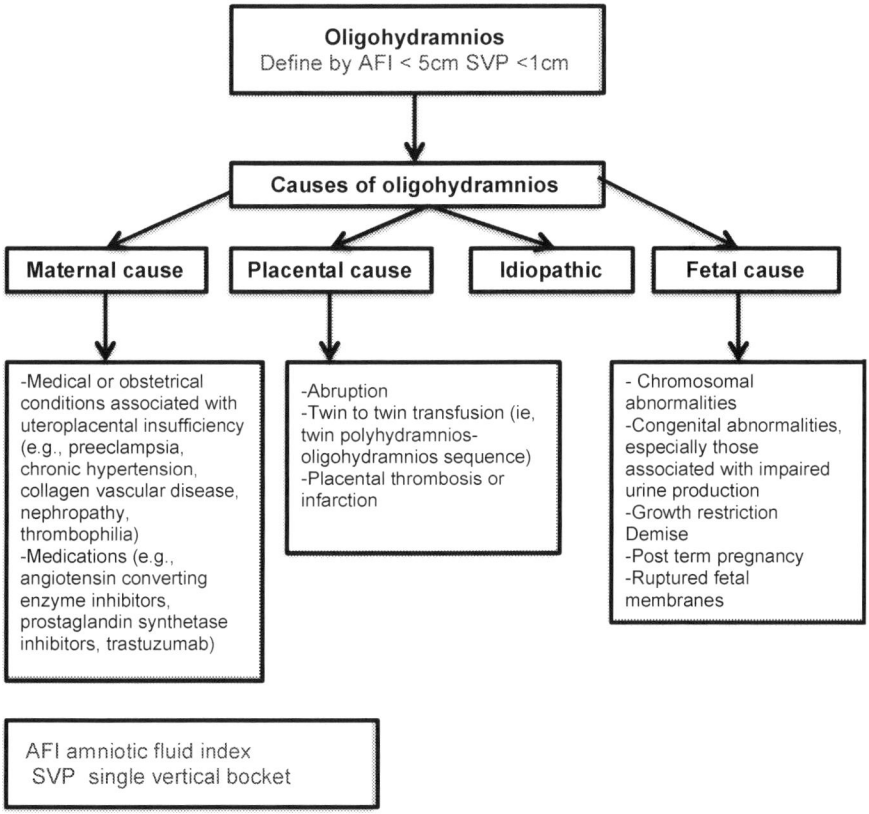

6.2 Management of oligohydramnios

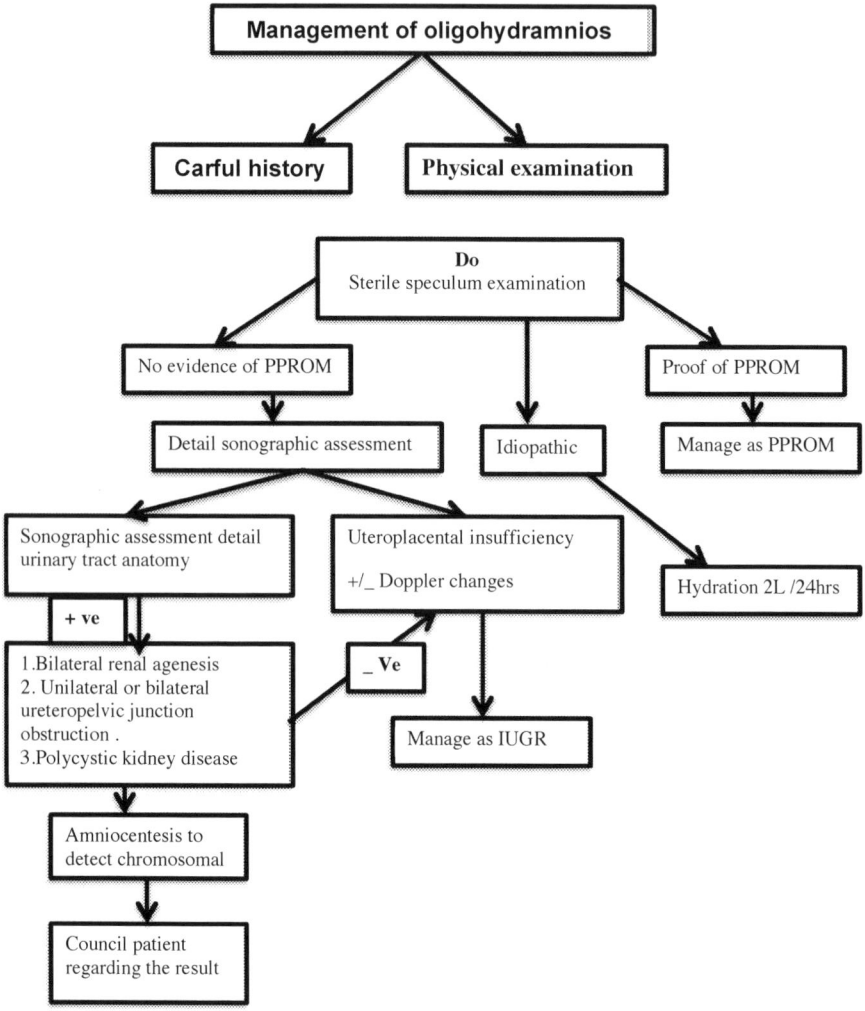

7 Polyhydramnios

7.1 Causes of oligohydramnios

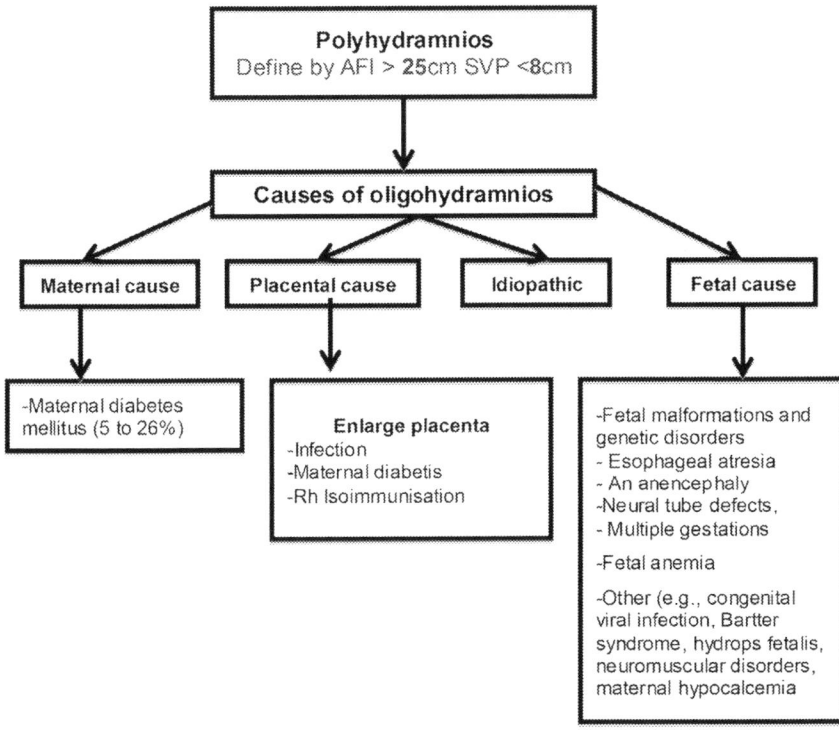

7.2 Management of polyhydramnios

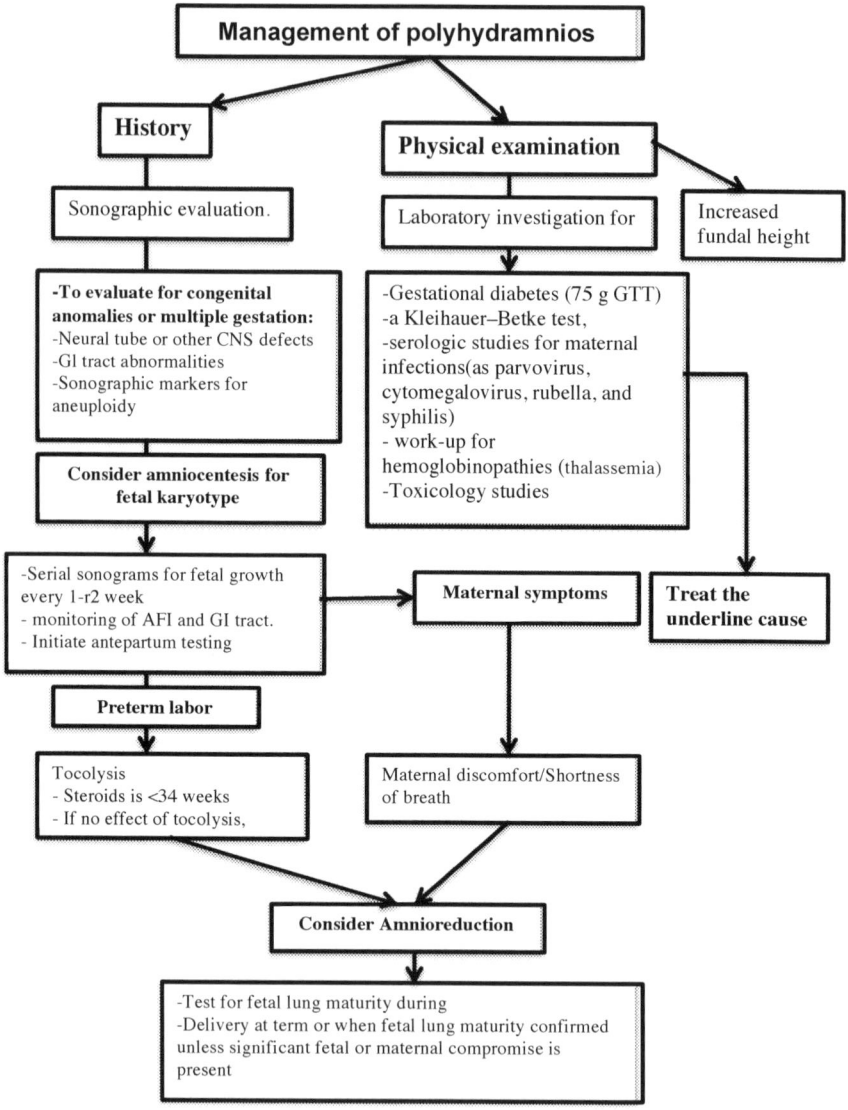

8 Intrauterine growth restriction

8.1 Management of IUGR

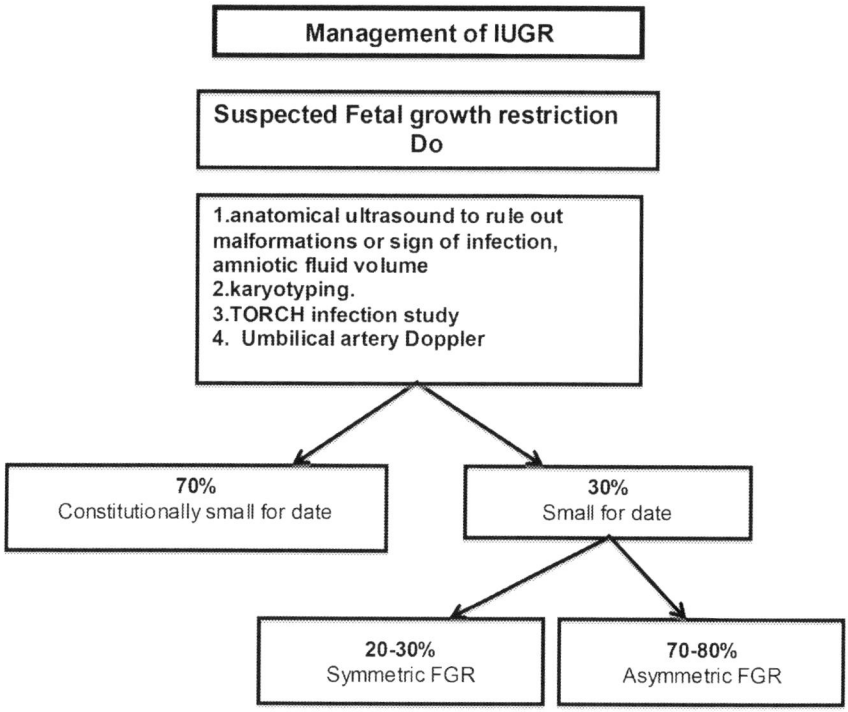

8.2 Asymmetrical IUGR

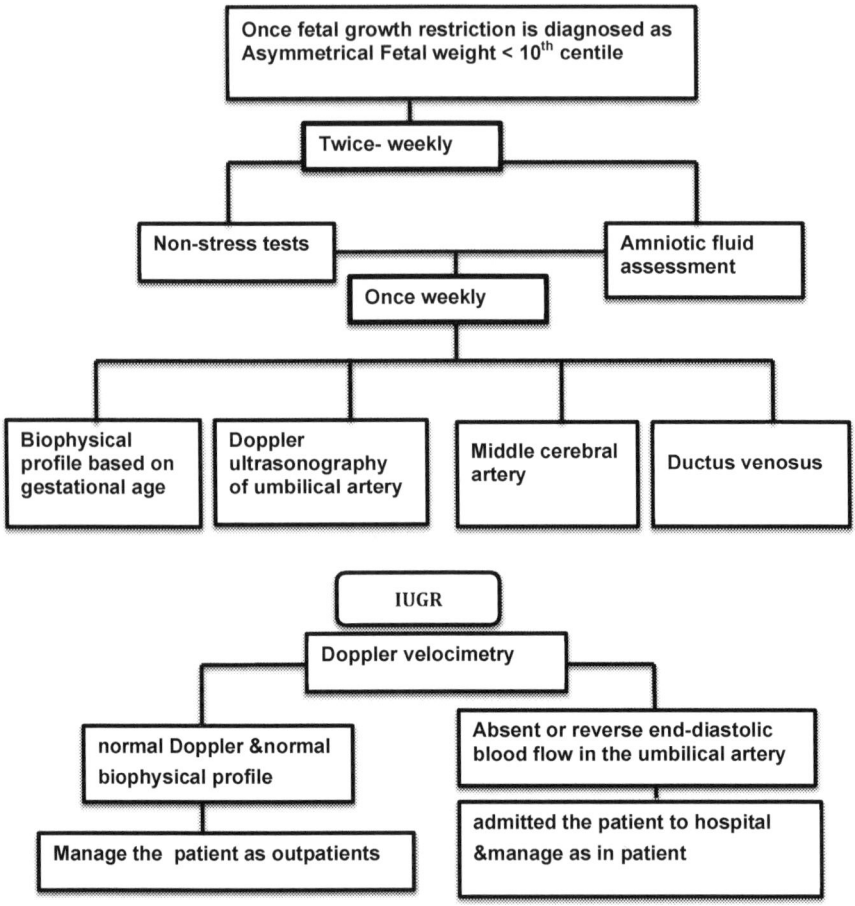

8.3 Management of Asymmetrical IUGR

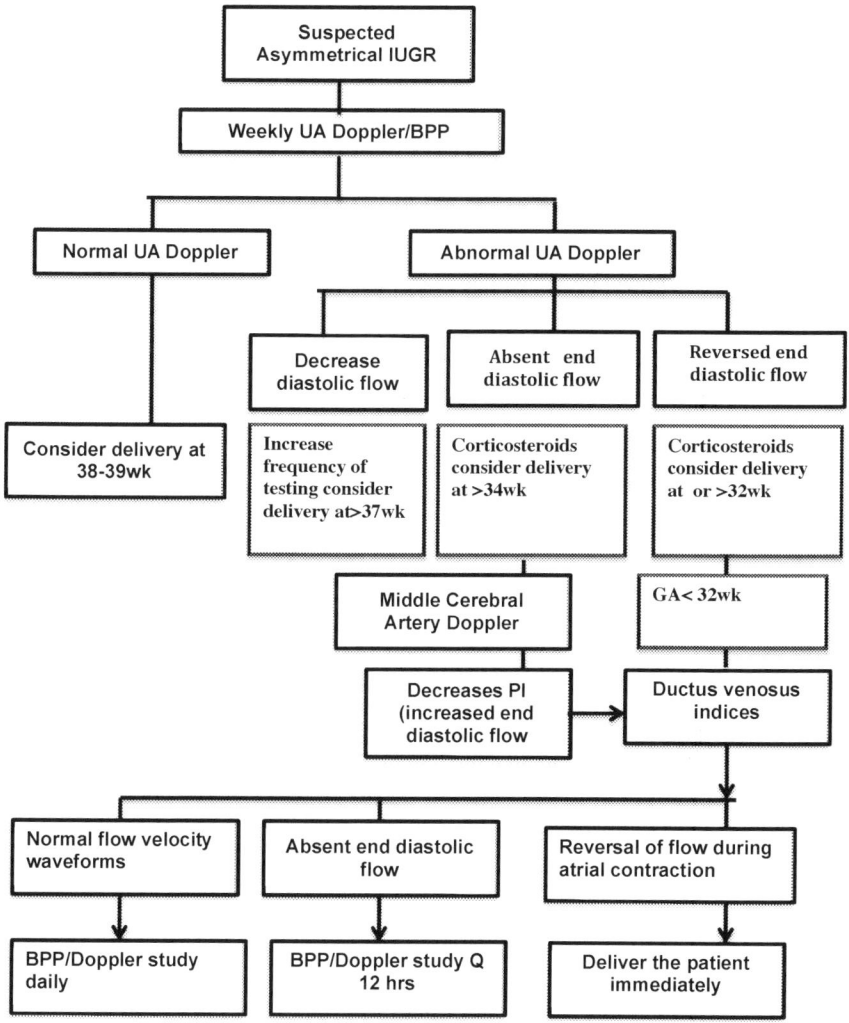

9 Urinary tract infections in pregnancy

9.1 Type of Urinary tract infections

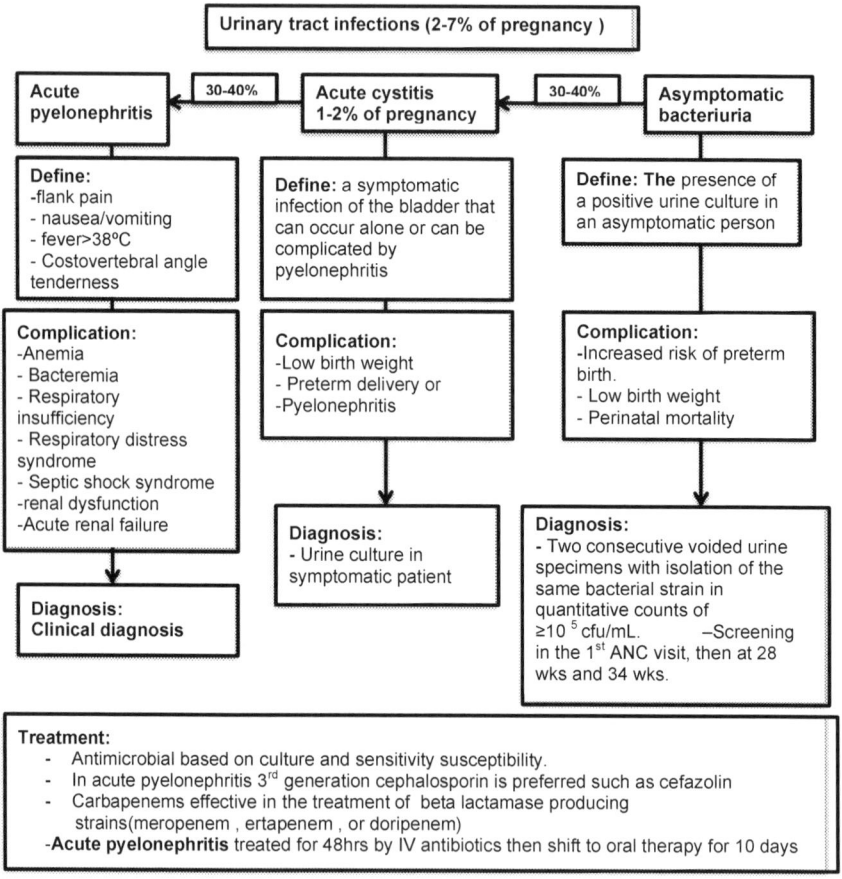

9.2 Management of Urinary tract infections

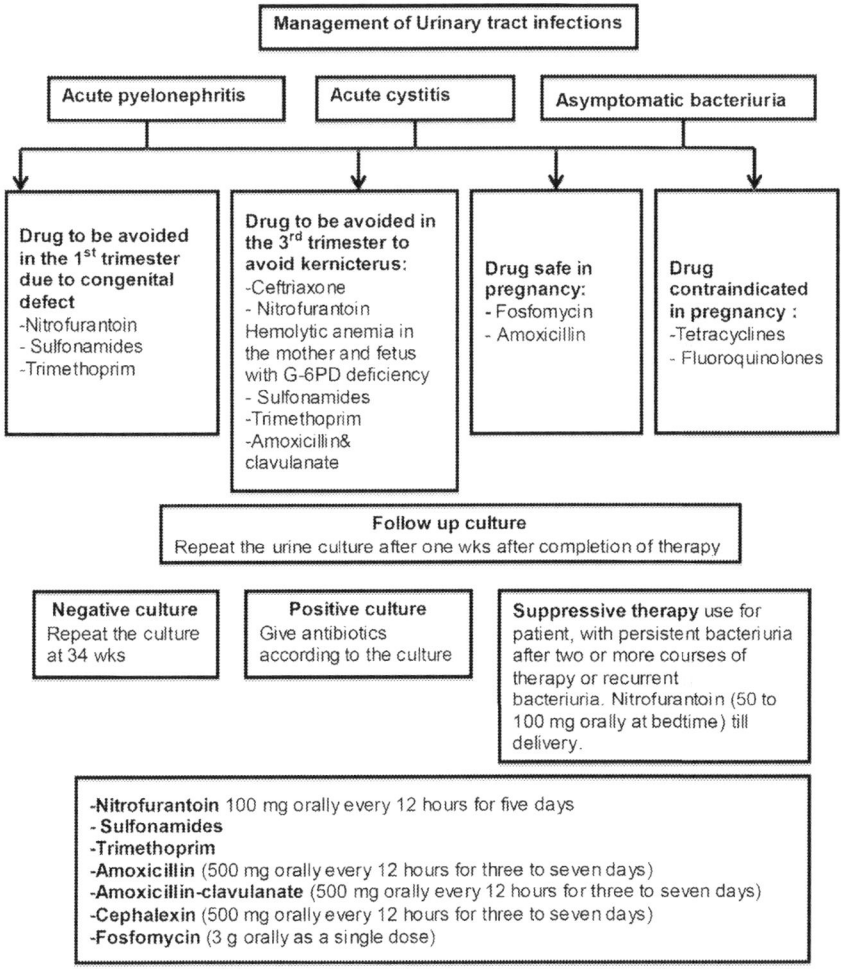

10 Intrahepatic cholestasis of pregnancy

10.1 Management of Intrahepatic cholestasis of pregnancy

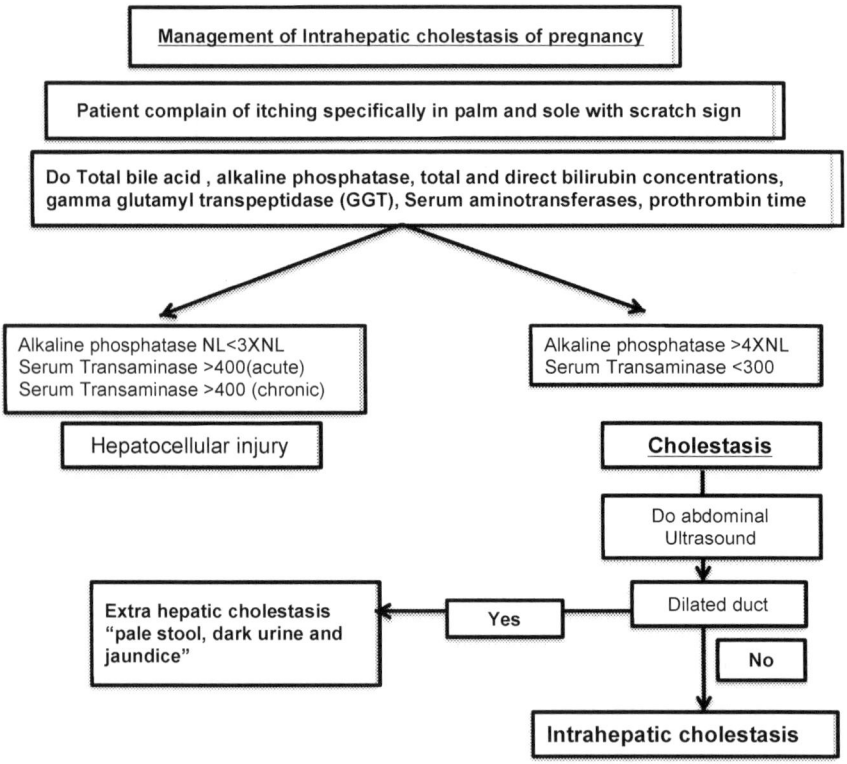

10.2 Management of Intrahepatic cholestasis of pregnancy2

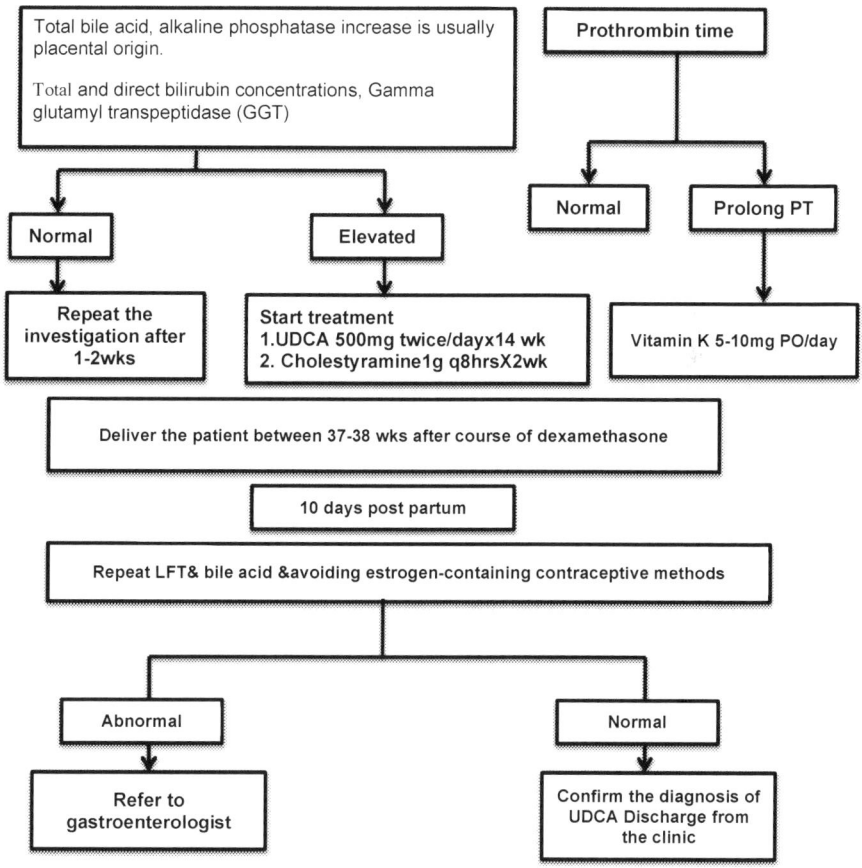

11 Varicella-zoster virus in pregnancy

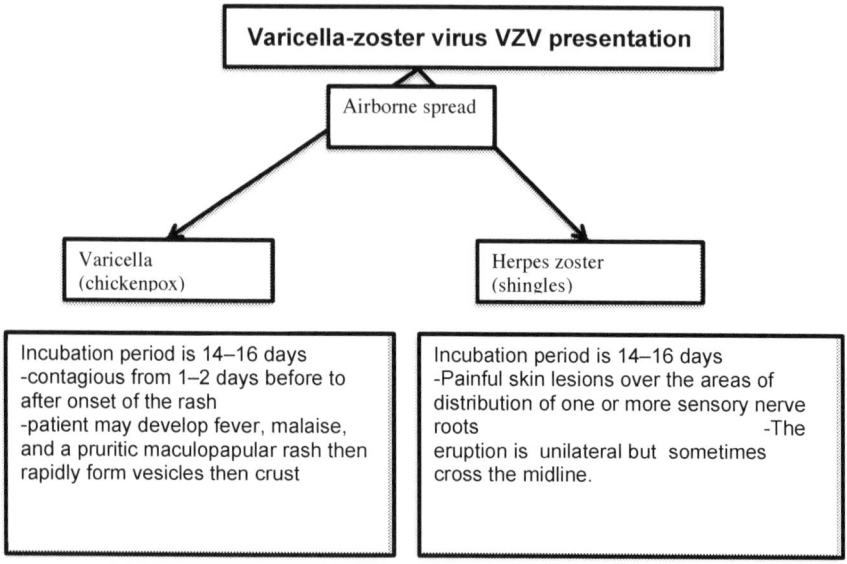

11.1 VZV complication

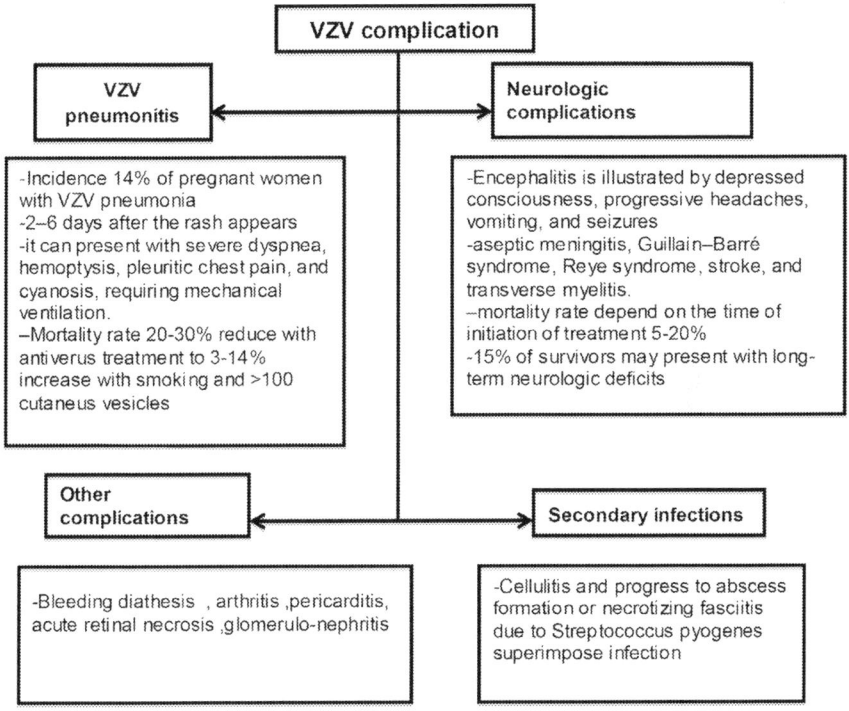

11.2 VZV diagnosis

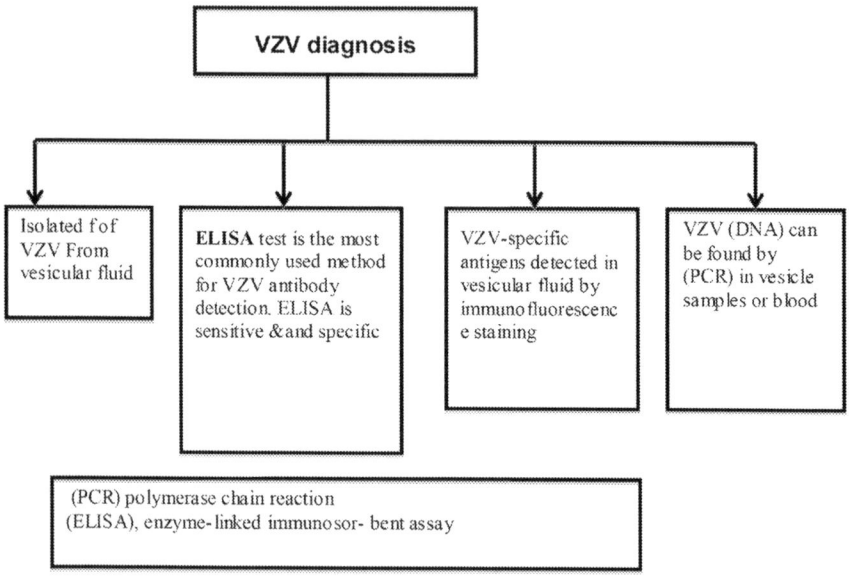

11.3 VZV Treatment

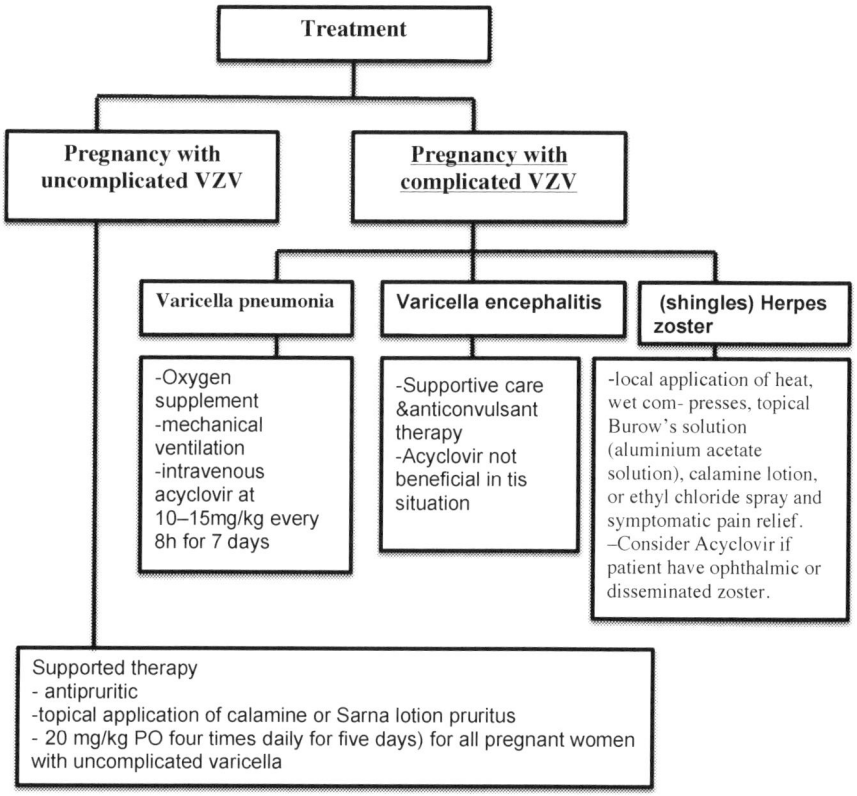

11.4 Management of VZV Exposure during pregnancy

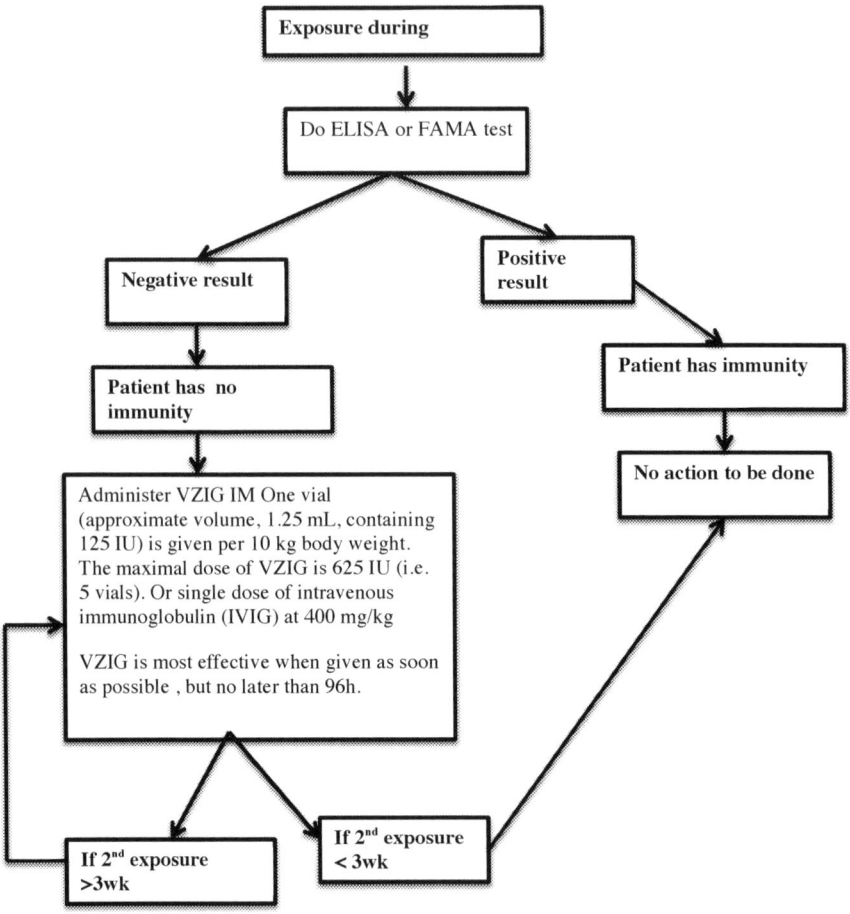

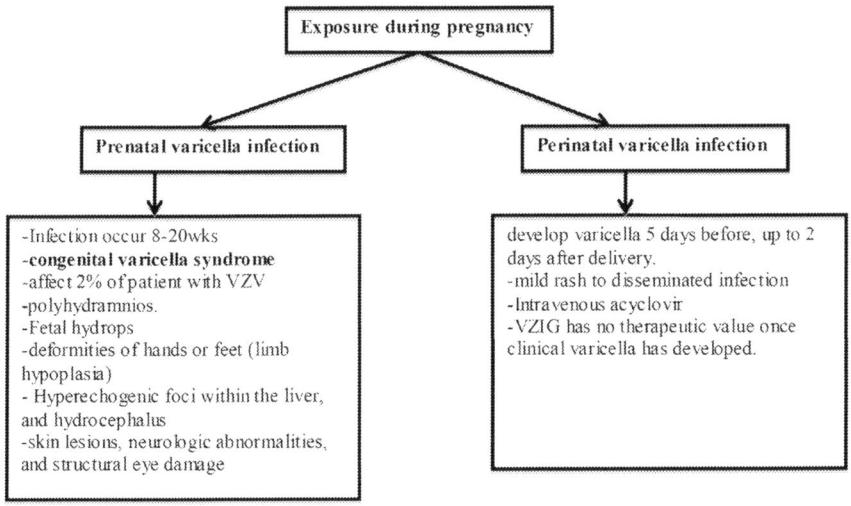
Exposure during pregnancy
Prenatal varicella infection
Perinatal varicella infection
-Infection occur 8-20wks
-congenital varicella syndrome
-affect 2% of patient with VZV
-polyhydramnios.
-Fetal hydrops
-deformities of hands or feet (limb hypoplasia)
- Hyperechogenic foci within the liver, and hydrocephalus
-skin lesions, neurologic abnormalities, and structural eye damage
develop varicella 5 days before, up to 2 days after delivery.
-mild rash to disseminated infection
-Intravenous acyclovir
-VZIG has no therapeutic value once clinical varicella has developed.

12 Toxoplasmosis and pregnancy

12.1 Toxoplasma infection during pregnancy

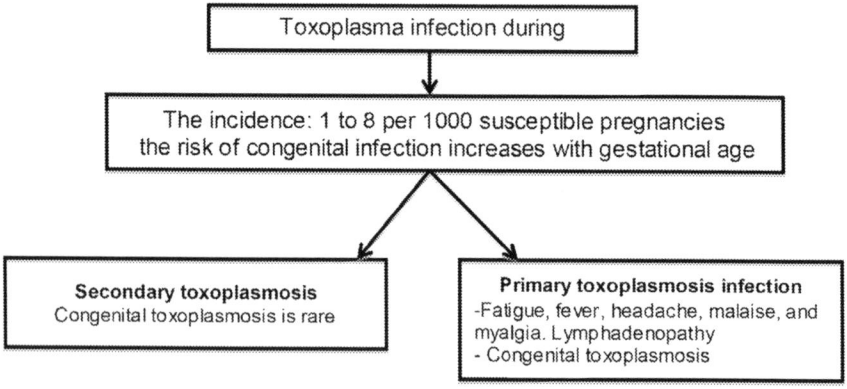

12.2 Toxoplasma infection diagnosis

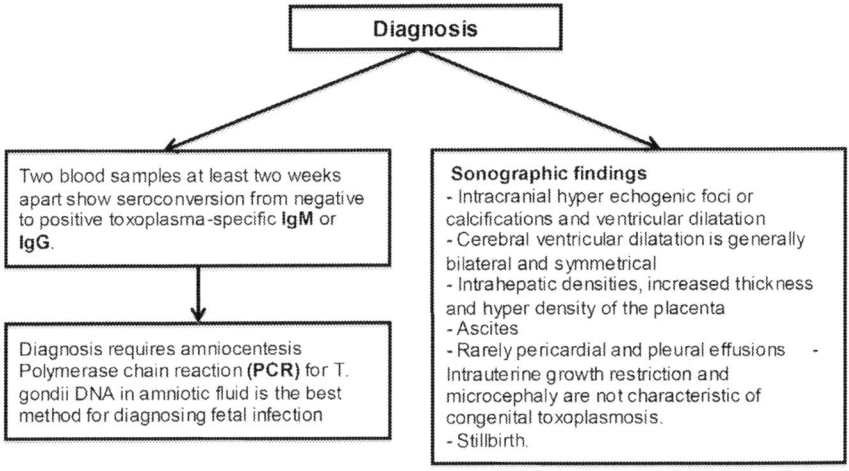

12.3 Tratment of Toxoplasma infection during pregnancy

Treatment

Infected during pregnancy are generally treated immediately with **spiramycin** (1 g orally every eight hours without food)
Pyrimethamine is a folic acid antagonist which can cause dose-related bone marrow suppression with resultant anemia, leukopenia, and thrombocytopenia
Sulfadiazine, can cause bone marrow suppression and reversible acute renal failure

Treatment

-Early treatment patients don't reduced the risk of intracranial lesions detected after birth, or of retinochoroiditis detected during infancy or mother-to-child transmission of infection -There is clear evidence that treatment reduce serious neurological sequelae or postnatal death in children with congenital toxoplasmosis

13 Gonorrheal infection in pregnancy

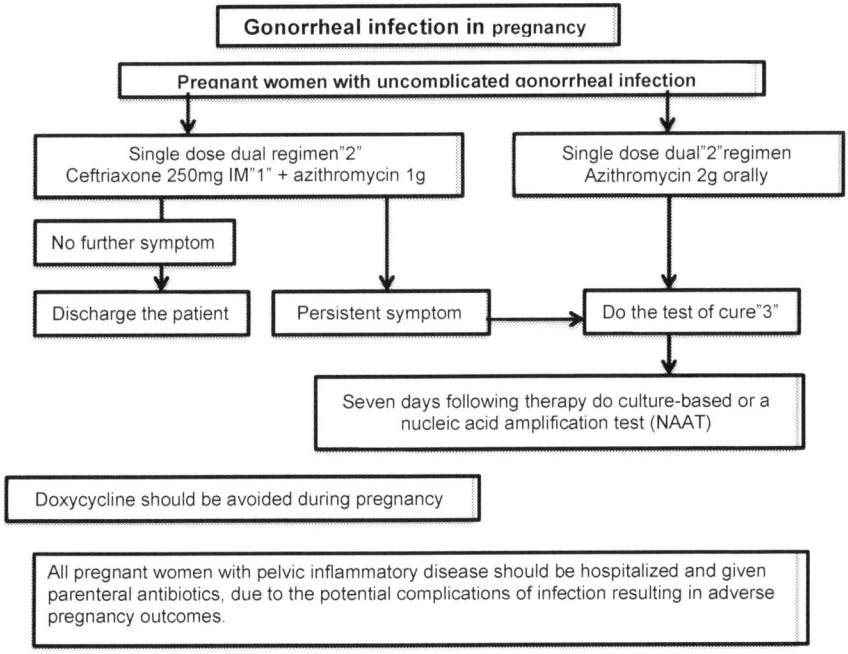

14 Hepatitis B during pregnancy

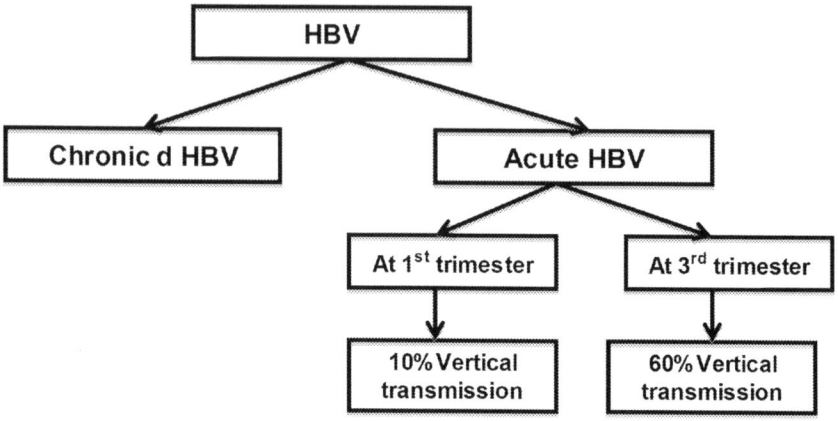

14.1 Management of acute HBV

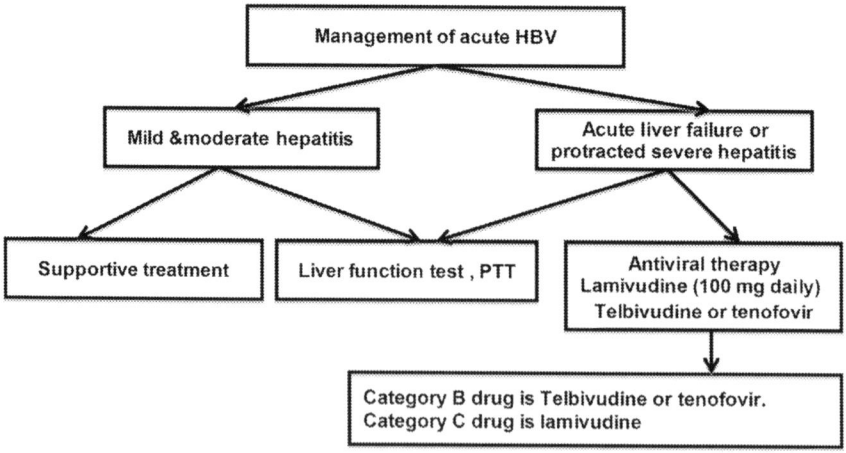

14.2 Chronic HBV

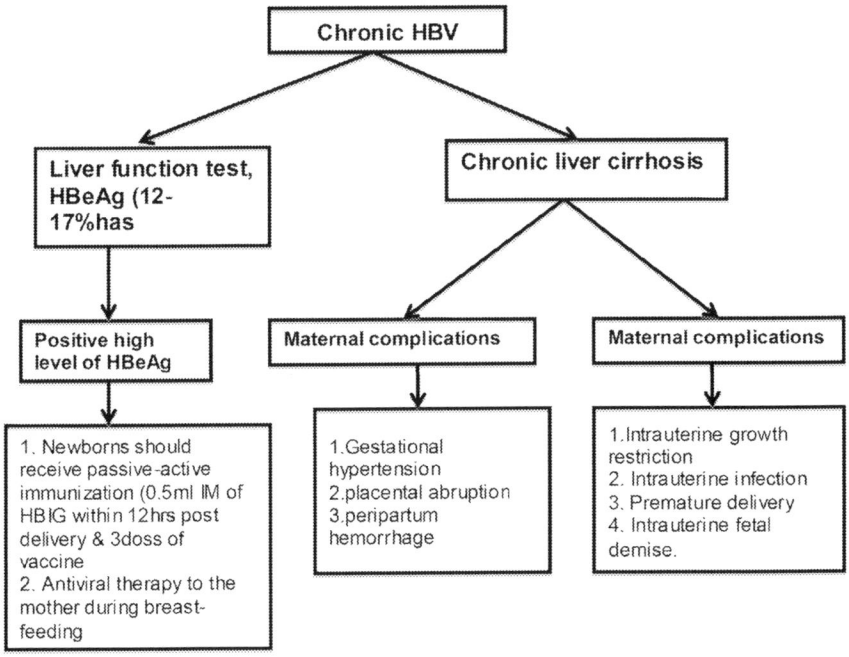

14.3 Breast-feeding in patient with HBV

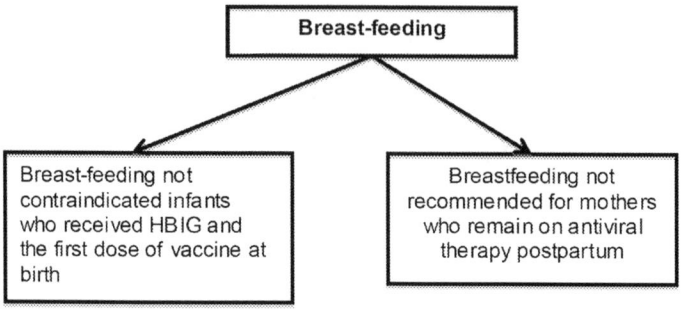

Dose of HBIG (0.06 ml/kg or 5.0 ml for adults) after accidental exposure to blood contaminated with hepatitis B

15 Cytomegalovirus infection in pregnancy

15.1 Cytomegalovirus infection (CMV)

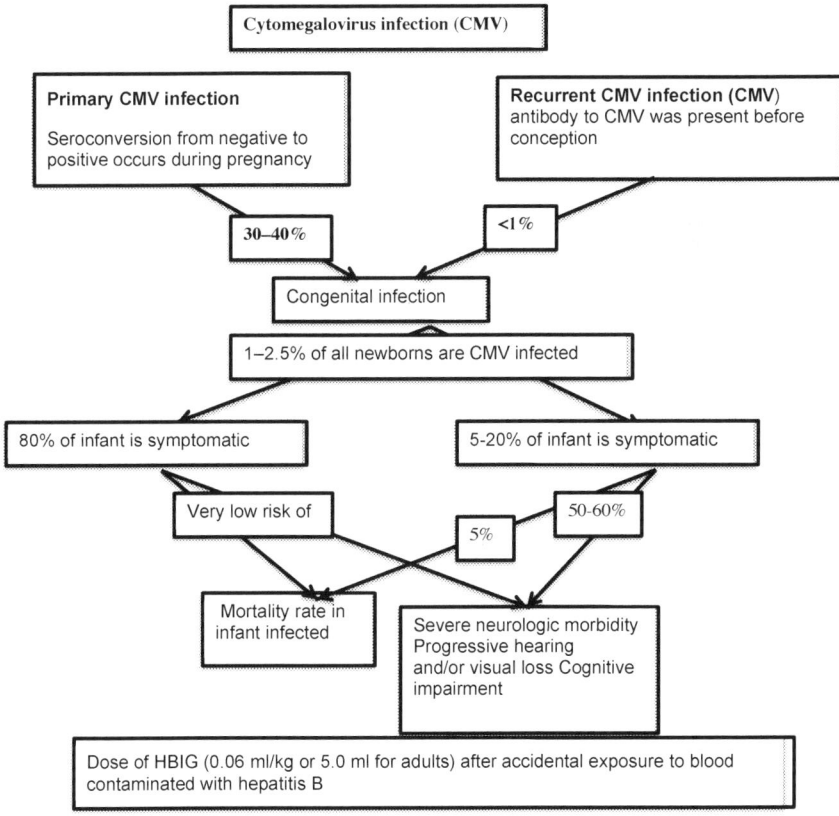

15.2 Maternal CMV infection

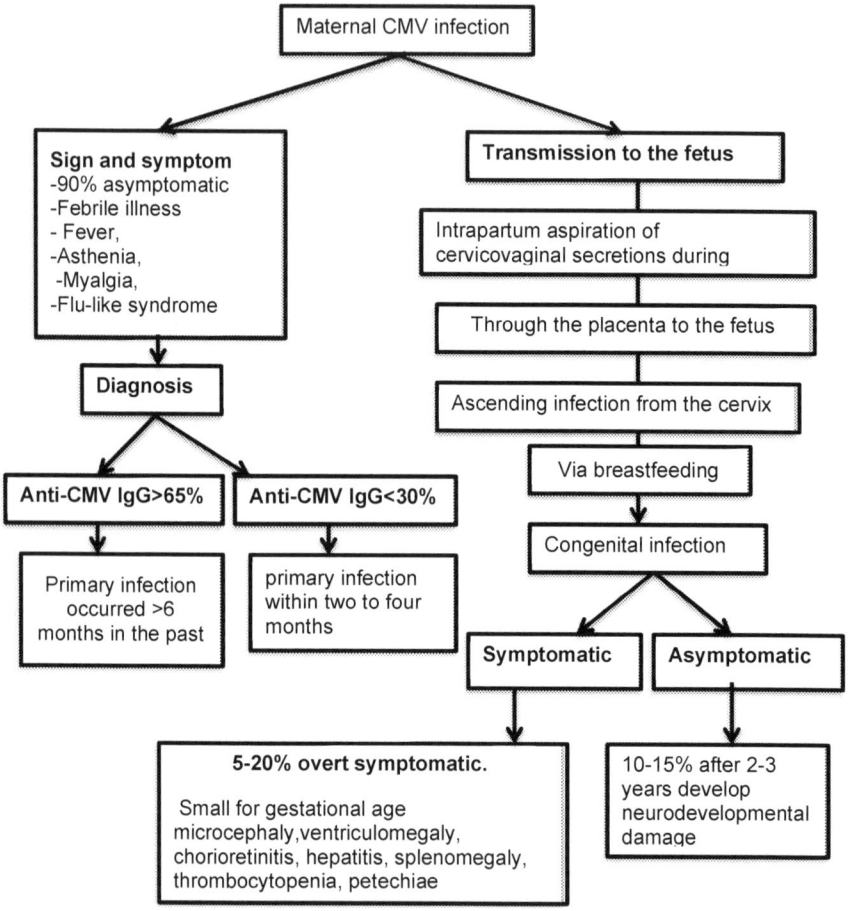

15.3 Prenatal diagnosis

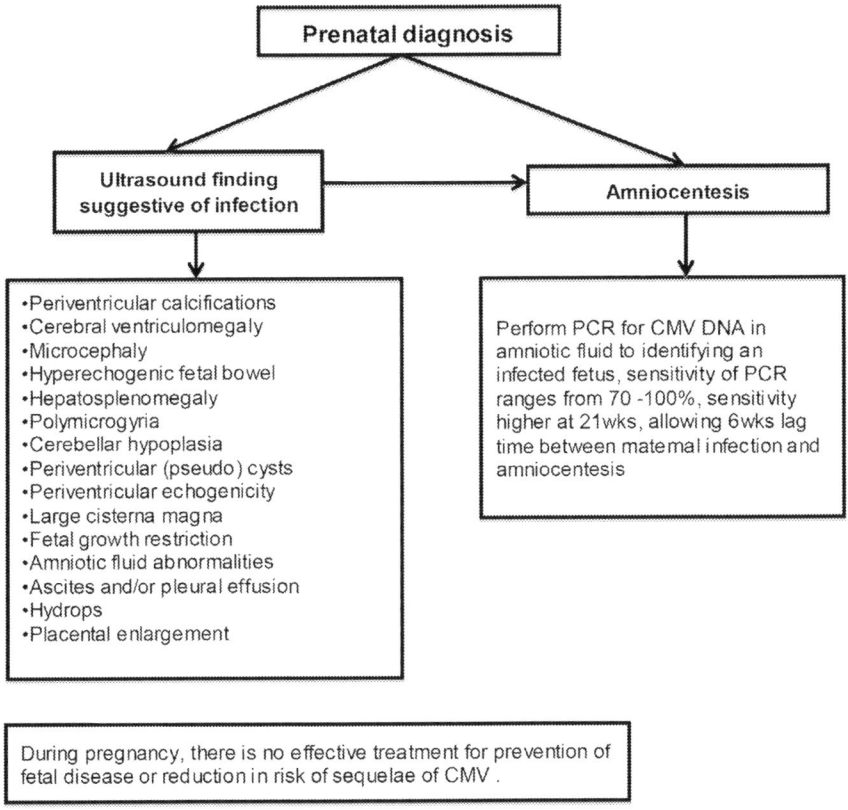

During pregnancy, there is no effective treatment for prevention of fetal disease or reduction in risk of sequelae of CMV .

16 Genital herpes simplex virus (HSV) infection

16.1 Genital herpes simplex virus (HSV) infection

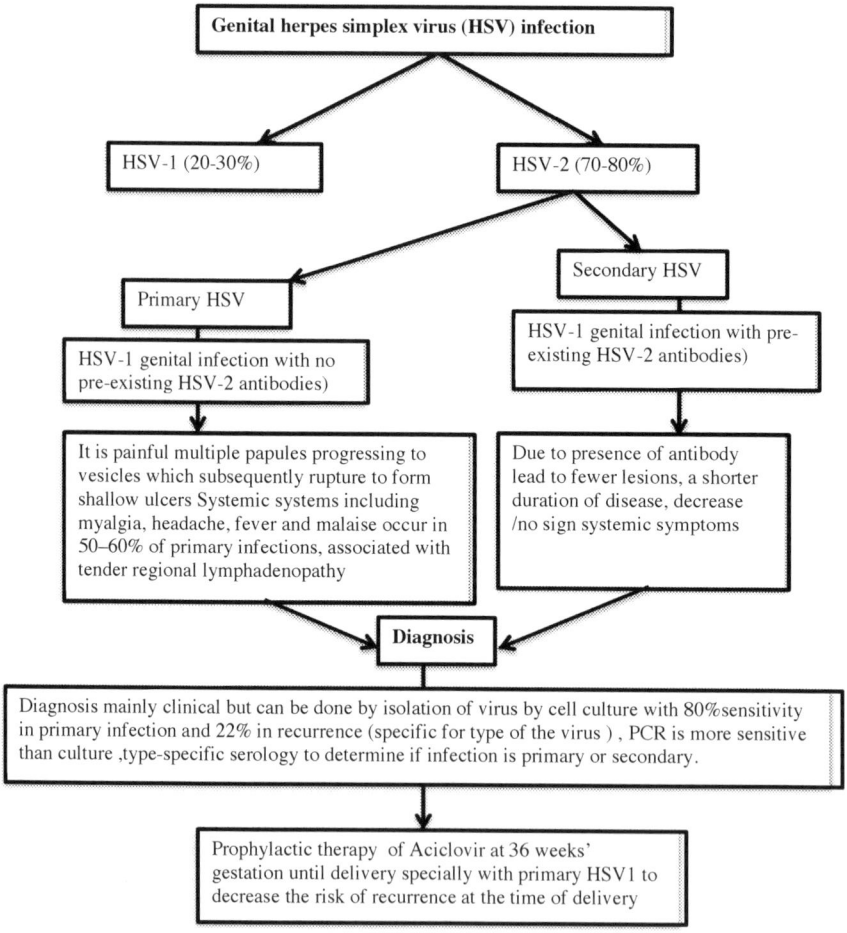

16.2 Genital Herpes during Labour or <34 weeks gestation

Genital Herpes during Labour or <34 weeks gestation

Primary

1. GUM Referral
2. Start oral/IV Acicovir – Explain the benefits and risks
3. Type specific HSV antibody testing

Aciclovir Regime

-200mgs 5 times daily/400mgs 3 times daily for 5 days -Disseminated HSV infection need IV Aciclovir

*Not licenced in pregnancy but no evidence of teratogenicity ***Avoid Aciclovir in <20 weeks**

Recurrent Episode

1. Antiviral Rx is rarely needed 2. Risk of transmission is small 3. Cultures to predict viral shedding at term is not indicated 4. C-Section is not indicated
5. C-Section & Prophylactic suppressive Aciclovir can be considered in women with herpetic lesions or co-infection with HIV

Abbreviations

GUM- Genito Urinary Medicine ARM- Artificial Rupture of Membranes HSV- Herpes Simplex Virus FSE- Fetal Scalp Electrode HIV- Human Immunodeficiency Virus FBS- Fetal Blood Sampling

16.3 Genital Herpes at >34 weeks

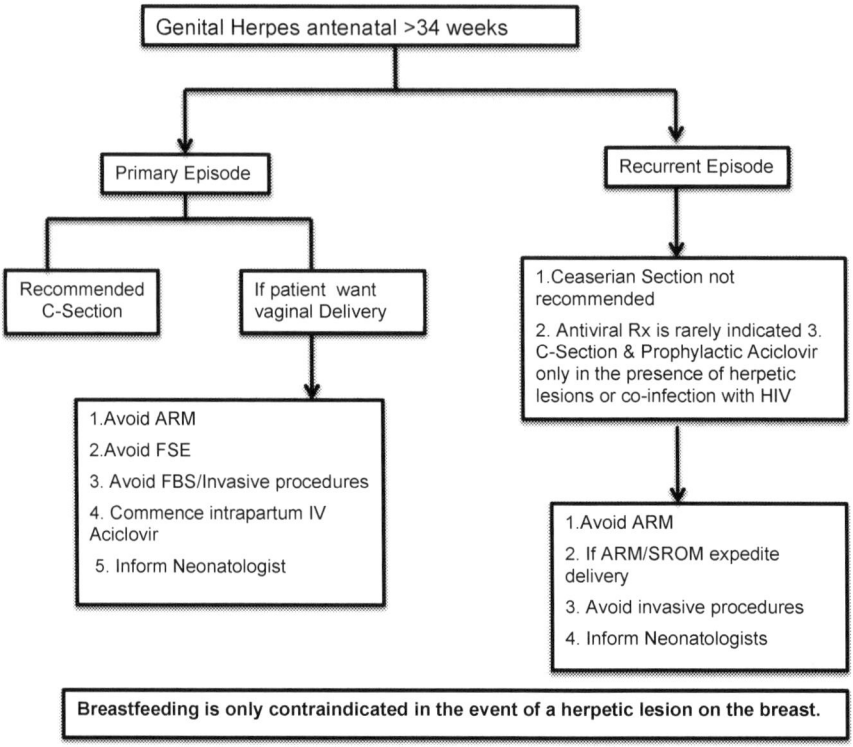

17 Parvovirus B19 infection

17.1 Parvovirus B19 infection

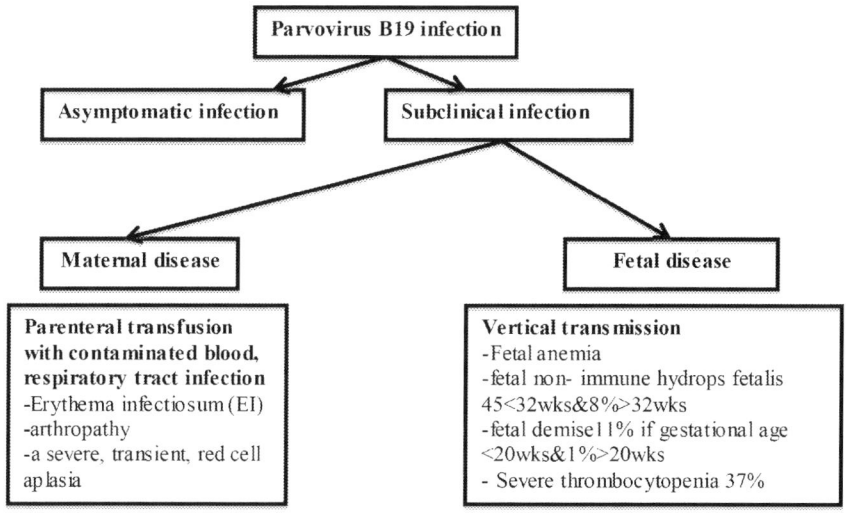

17.2 Parvovirus B19 infection diagnosia

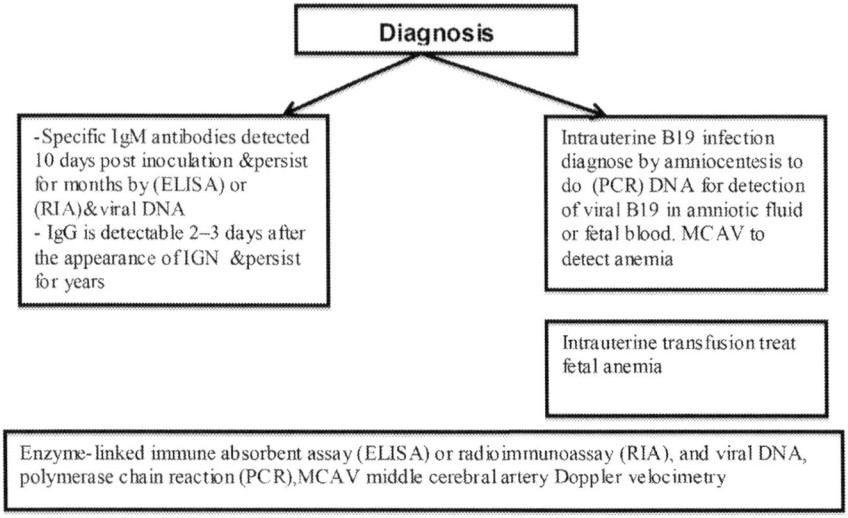

18 Syphilis in pregnancy

18.1 Stages of Syphilis during pregnancy

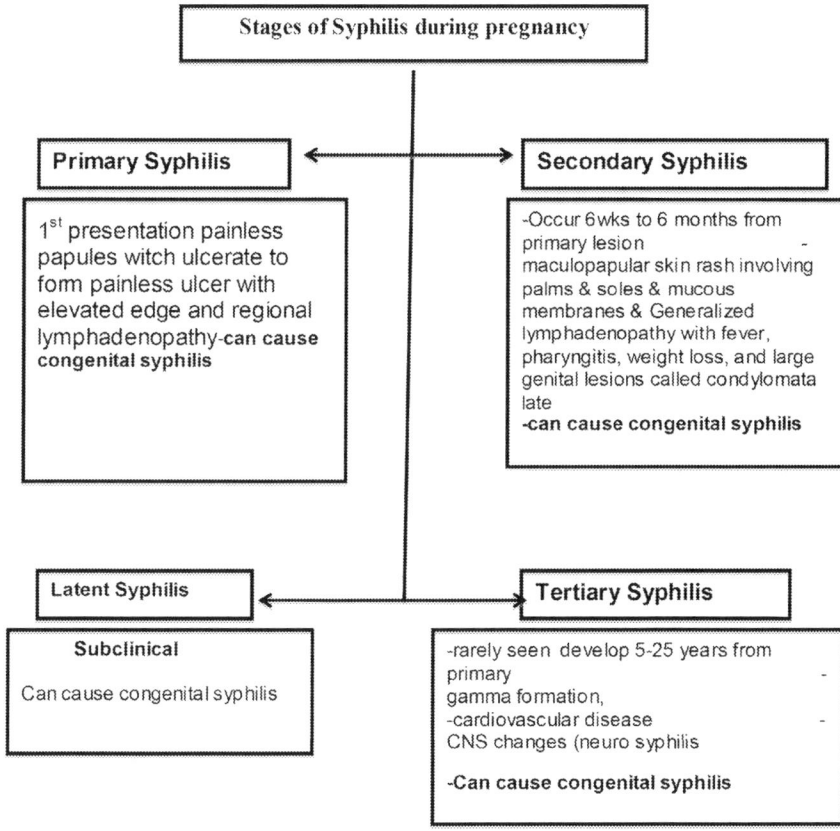

18.2 Syphilis complicating pregnancy

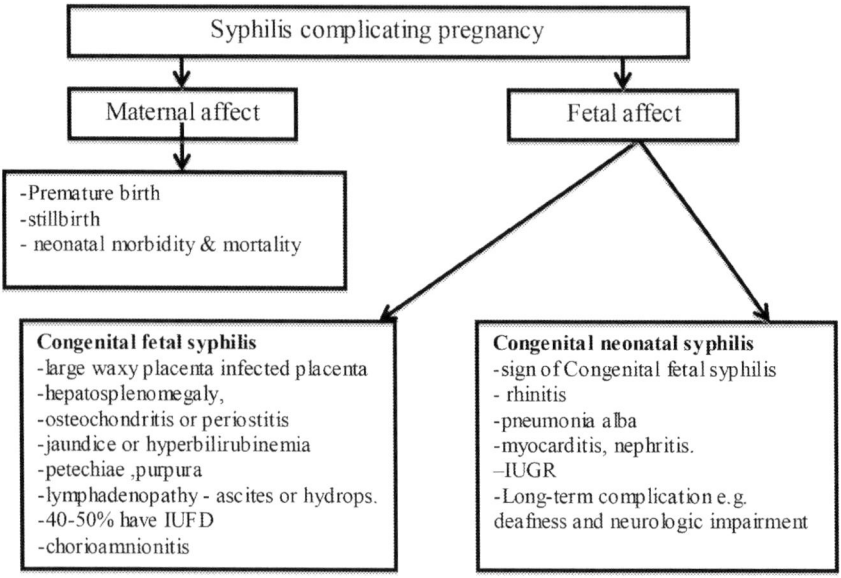

18.3 Syphilis Diagnosis

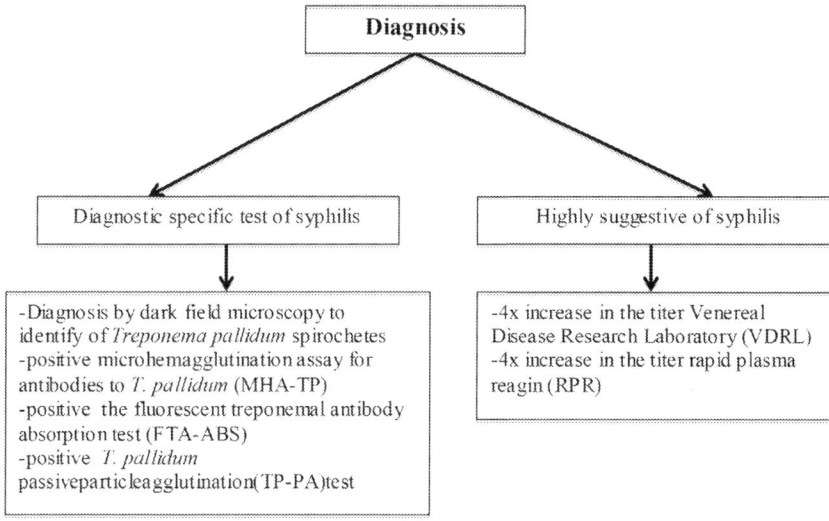

18.4 Management of syphilis in pregnancy

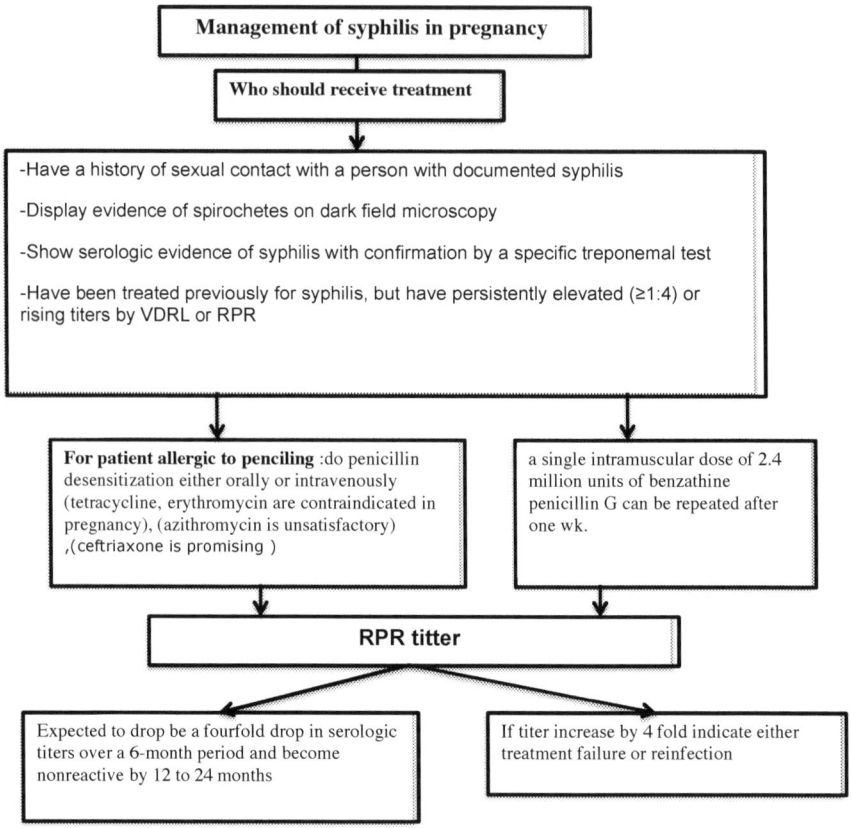

19 Sickle cell disease with pregnancy

19.1 Prepregnancy evaluation of sickle cell disease

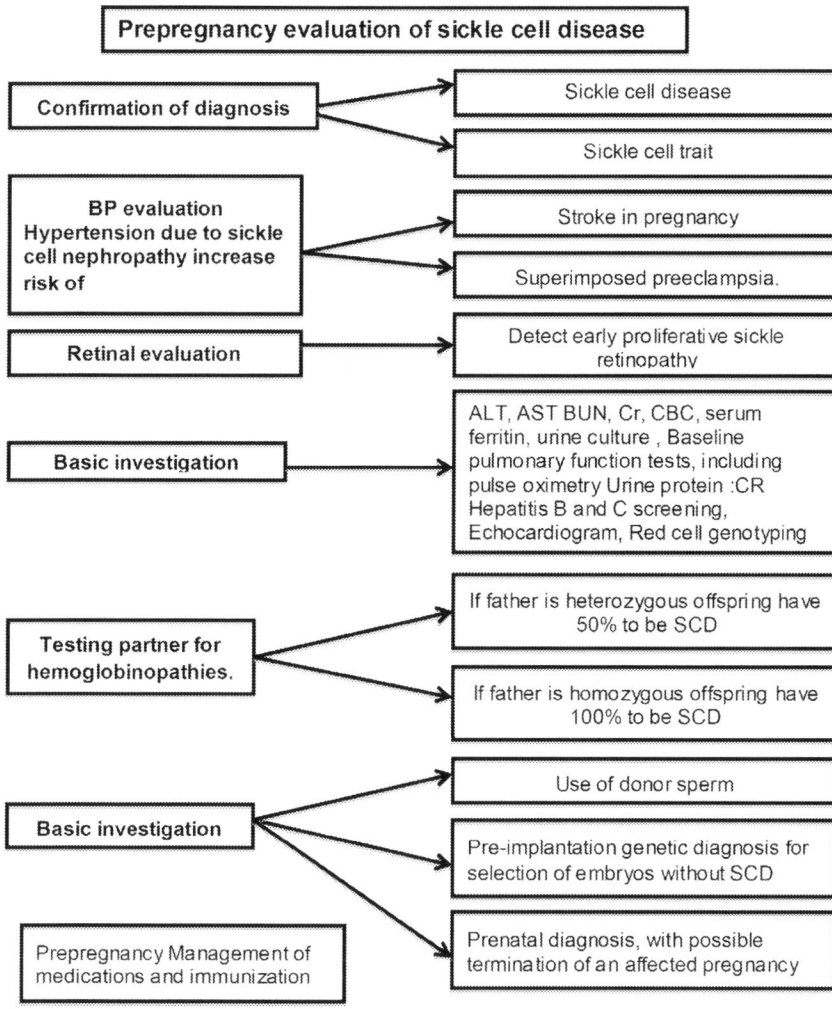

19.2 Prepregnancy Management of medications & immunization in sickle cell disease patient

Prepregnancy Management of medications & immunization

Immunization	Give the vaccine for polyvalent pneumococcal; Haemophilus influenza type B, and meningococcal vaccines avoid pregnancy for four weeks after administration of a live vaccine.
Folic acid	Recommended dose 5mg /day
Iron chelators	Discontinue iron chelation therapy once conceive
Hydroxyurea	Discontinue hydroxyurea three months before conception
ACE inhibitors and ARBs	Discontinue this medication because it is teratogenicity
Prophylactic penicillin	penicillin therapy may be continued during pregnancy
Analgesia	NSAIDs avoided after 30 wks because of the risk of premature closure of ductus arteriosus

19.3 Risk of sickle cell disease on pregnancy

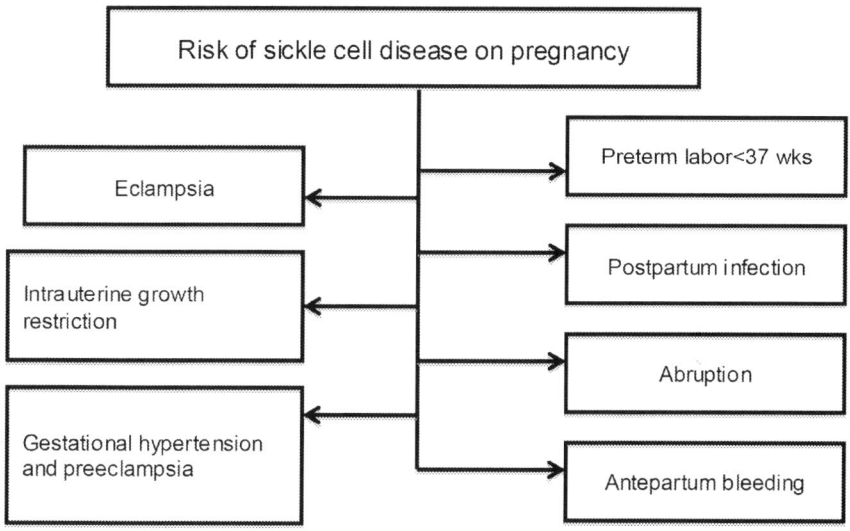

19.4 Prenatal care of sickle cell disease "HbSS, HbSC, HbS/beta-thal

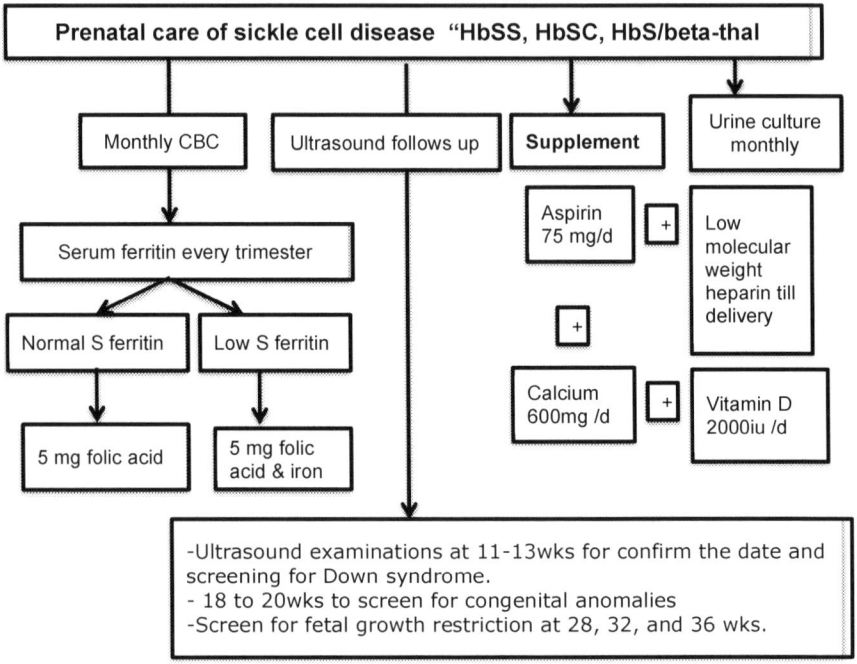

19.5 Management of complication

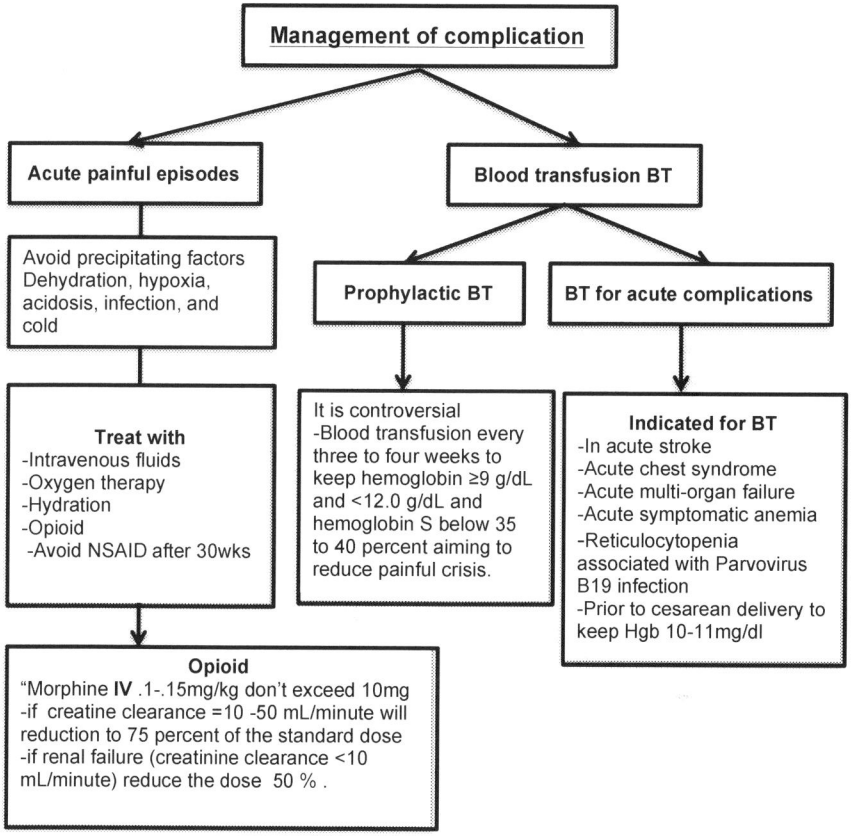

20 Hypothyroidism

20.1 Hypothyroidism in preconception

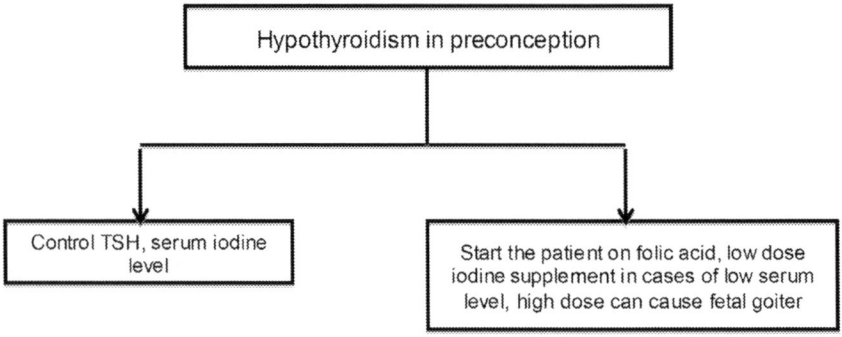

20.2 Thyroid disease in pregnancy

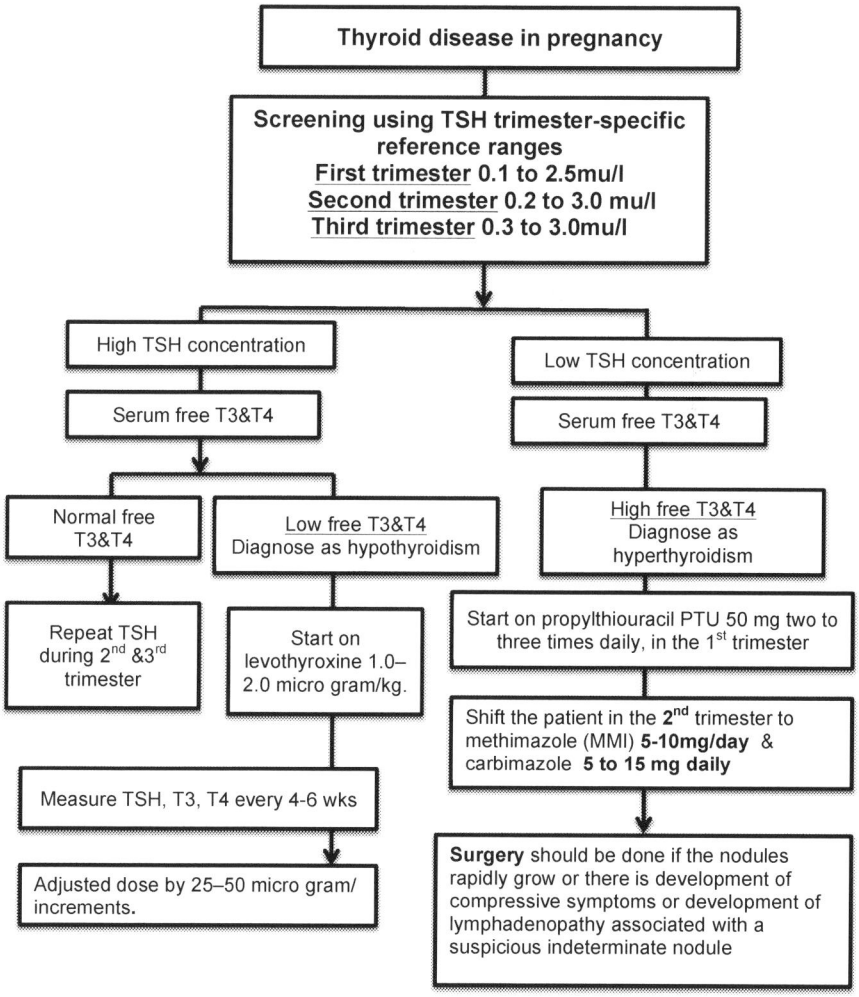

21 Diabetes

21.1 Gestational diabetes

Gestational diabetes

Preconception visit

1.A family history of diabetes, especially in first degree relatives

2.Prepregnancy weight ≥110 percent of ideal body weight or body mass index >30 kg/m 2 or excessive gestational weight gain

3.Age >25 years

4.Previous delivery of a baby >9 pounds [4.1 kg]

5.Personal history of impaired glucose tolerance

6.Member of an ethnic group with higher than the background rate of type 2 diabetes (eg, Hispanic-American, African-American, Native American, South or East Asian, Pacific Islander).

7.Previous unexplained perinatal loss or birth of a malformed infant

8.Maternal birthweight >9 pounds [4.1 kg] or <6 pounds [2.7 kg]

9.Glycosuria at the first prenatal visit

10.Polycystic ovary syndrome

11.Current use of glucocorticoids

12.Essential hypertension or pregnancy-related hypertension

13.Metabolic syndrome

If the patient has one or more risk factor screen for gestational diabetis A1C

21.2 screen for gestational diabetis

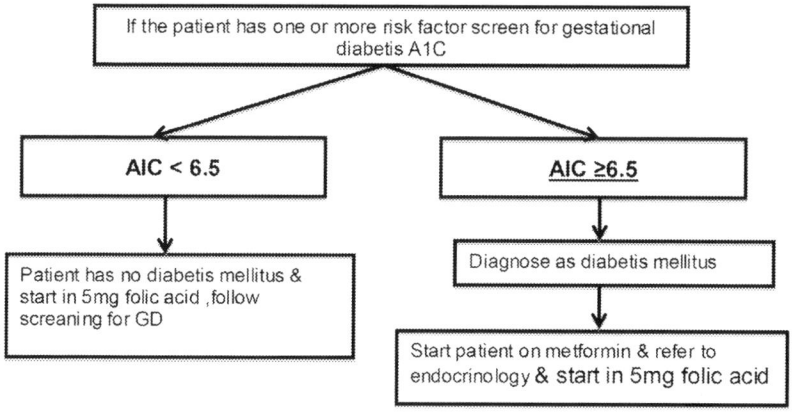

Normal value for BSP FBS<92 mg/dL (5.1 mmol/L) 2hrs postprandial 2-h <140 mg/dl (7.7 mmol)

75g GTT normal value (one abnormal value will consider the patient gestational diabetis
Fasting plasma glucose ≥92 mg/dL [5.1 mmol/L], **one hour** ≥180 mg/dL (10.0 mmol/L) **two hour** ≥153 mg/dL (8.5 mmol/L)

21.3 Follow up of gestational diabetis

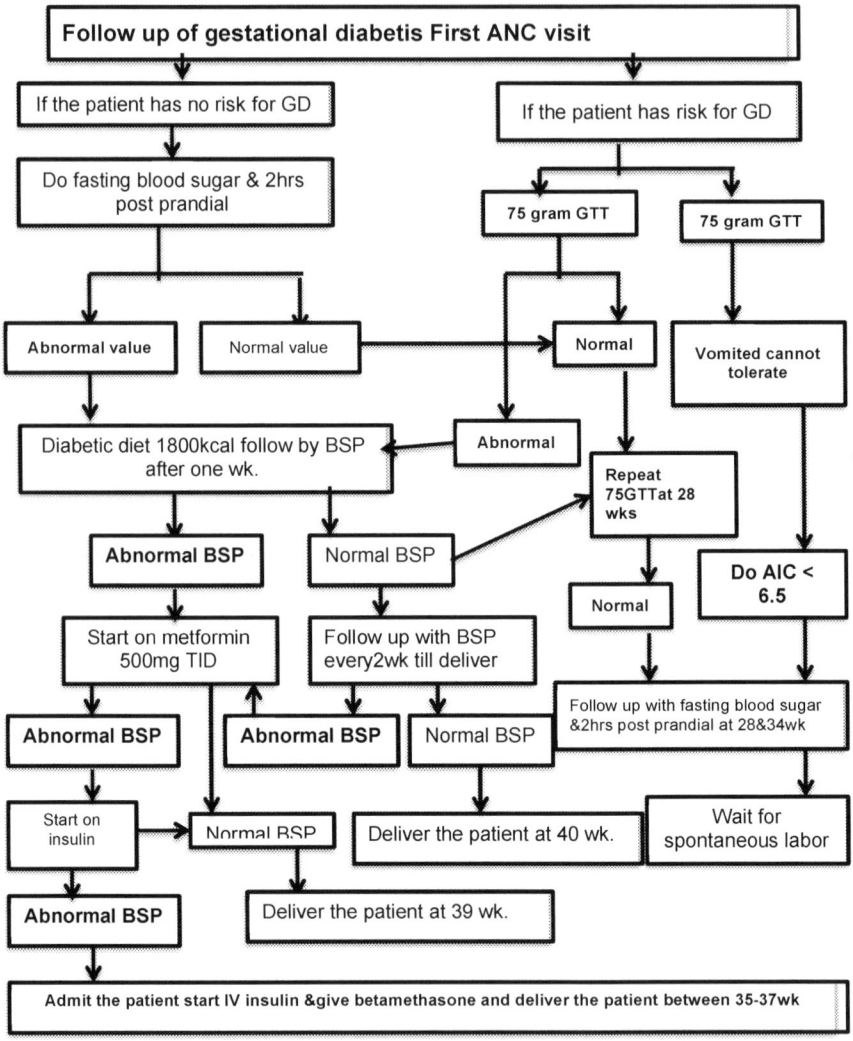

22 Preconception type 1&type 2 diabetes mellitus

22.1 Preconception management of type 1&type 2 diabetes mellitus

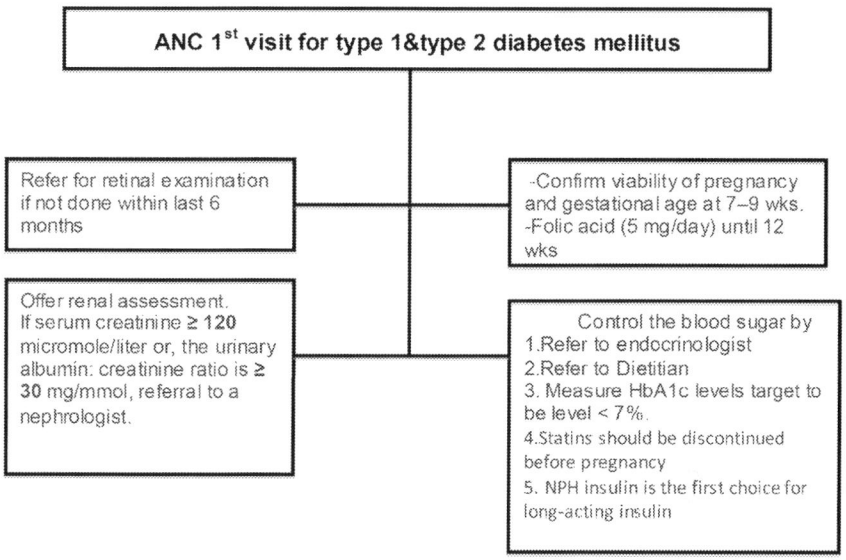

22.2 Preconception management of type 1&type 2 diabetes mellitus

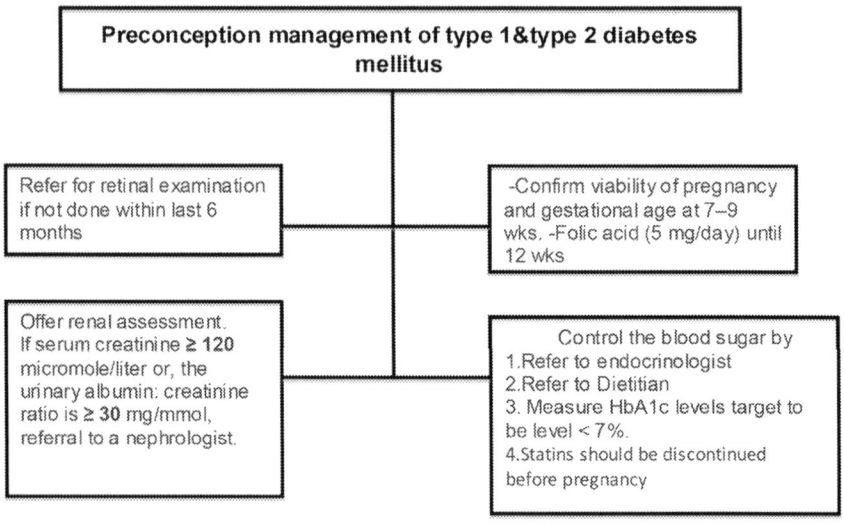

22.3 ANC follow up for type 1&type 2 diabetes mellitus

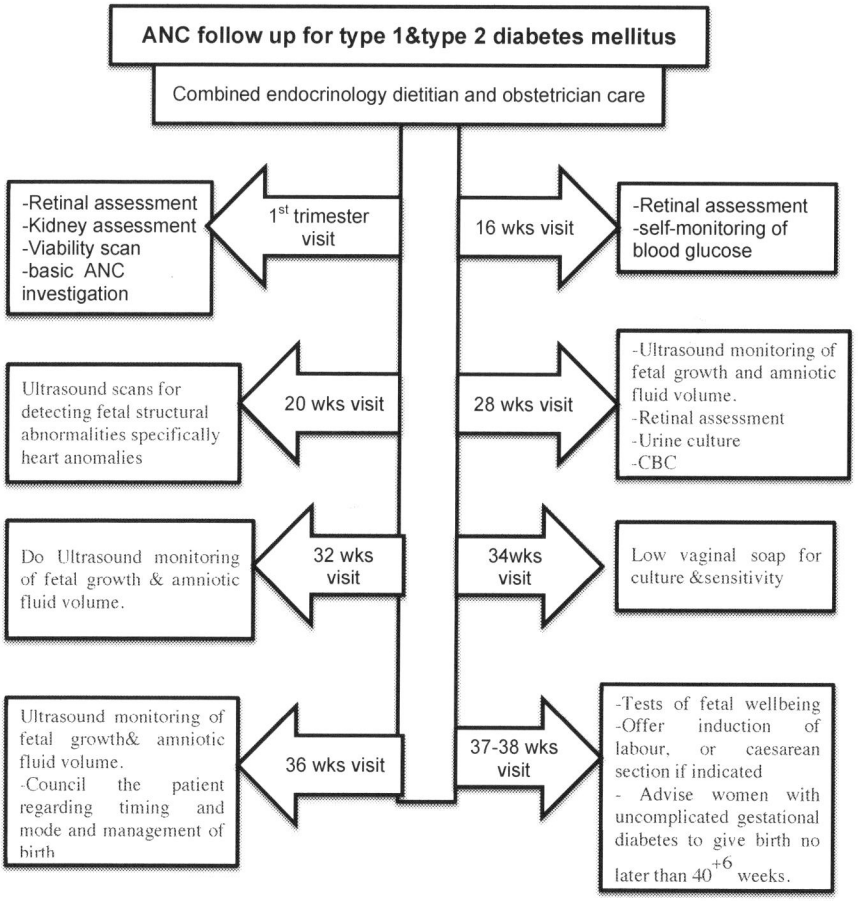

22.4 Intrapartum care for patient with diabetis mellitus

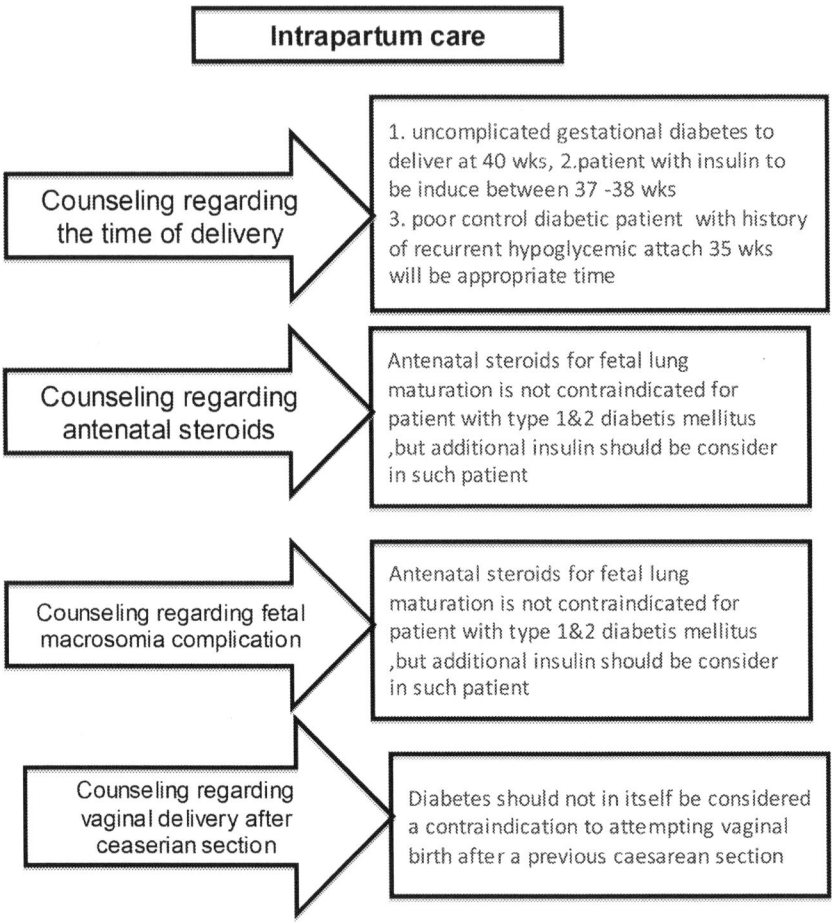

22.5 Post natal care with diabetis mellitus type1&2

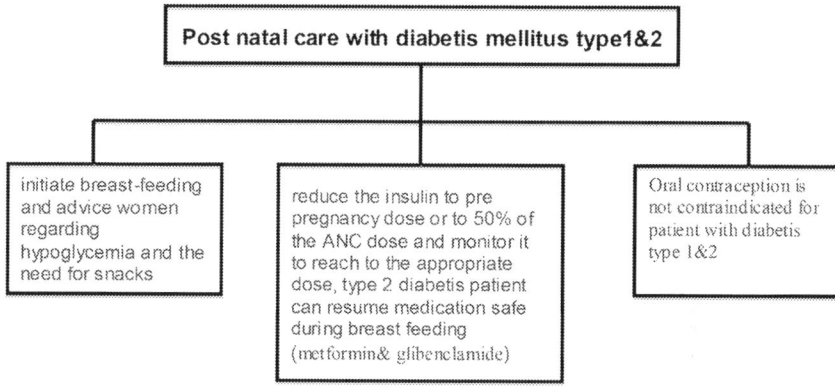

23 Hypertension in pregnancy

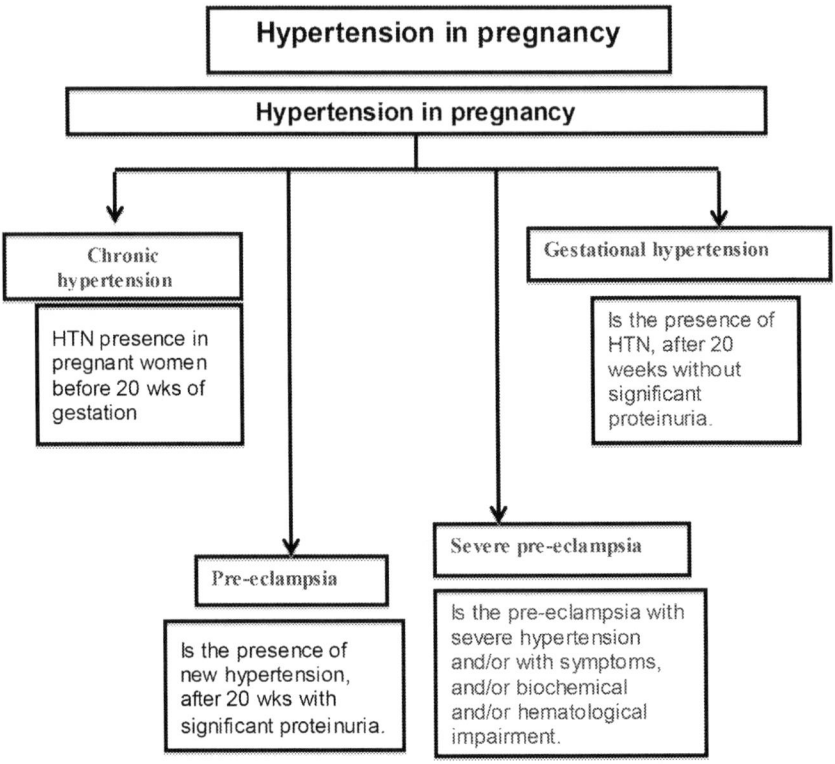

23.1 Risk factors for pre-eclampsia

The risk factors for pre-eclampsia

1.Hypertensive disease during a previous pregnancy

2.Chronic kidney disease

3.Autoimmune disease such as systemic lupus erythematosus or antiphospholipid syndrome

4.Type 1 or type 2 diabetes

5.Chronic hypertension.

Advise women at high risk of pre-eclampsia to take 81 mg of aspirin

-Women with chronic HTN advice to stop angiotensin-converting enzyme (ACE) because of risk of congenital anomalies

23.2 HTN disease in pregnancy

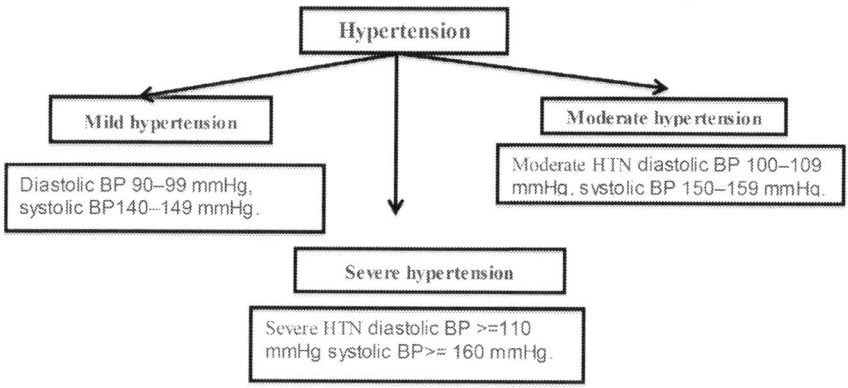

23.3 Chronic hypertension in pregnancy

Management of chronic HTN during pregnancy

ANC follow up

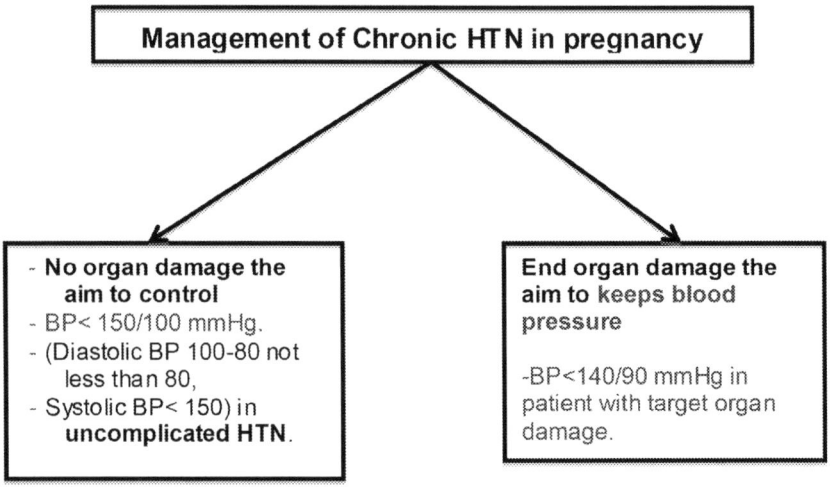

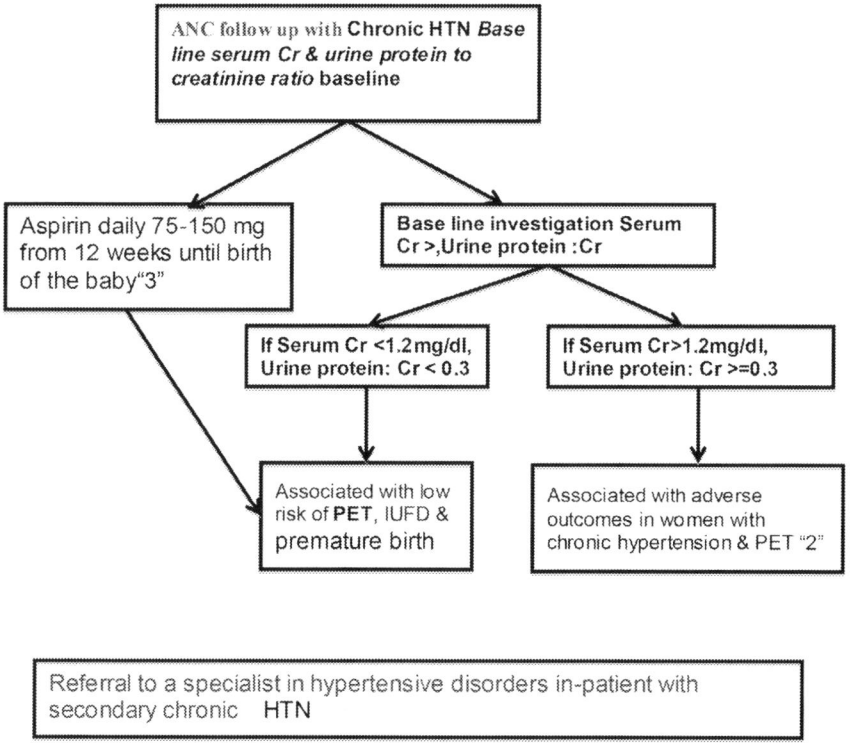
ANC follow up with Chronic HTN Base line serum Cr & urine protein to creatinine ratio baseline
Aspirin daily 75-150 mg from 12 weeks until birth of the baby"3"
Base line investigation Serum Cr >,Urine protein :Cr
If Serum Cr <1.2mg/dl, Urine protein: Cr < 0.3
If Serum Cr>1.2mg/dl, Urine protein: Cr >=0.3
Associated with low risk of PET, IUFD & premature birth
Associated with adverse outcomes in women with chronic hypertension & PET "2"
Referral to a specialist in hypertensive disorders in-patient with secondary chronic HTN

23.4 Antihypertensive drug during pregnancy

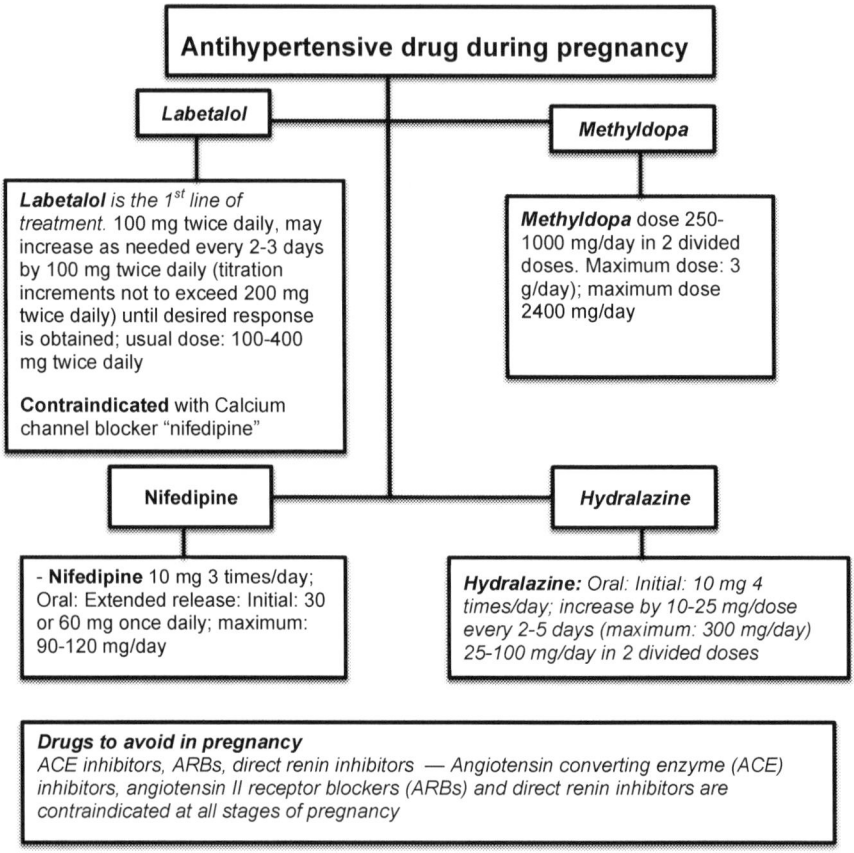

Drugs to avoid in pregnancy
ACE inhibitors, ARBs, direct renin inhibitors — Angiotensin converting enzyme (ACE) inhibitors, angiotensin II receptor blockers (ARBs) and direct renin inhibitors are contraindicated at all stages of pregnancy

23.5 BP target in treatment of HTN disease in pregnancy

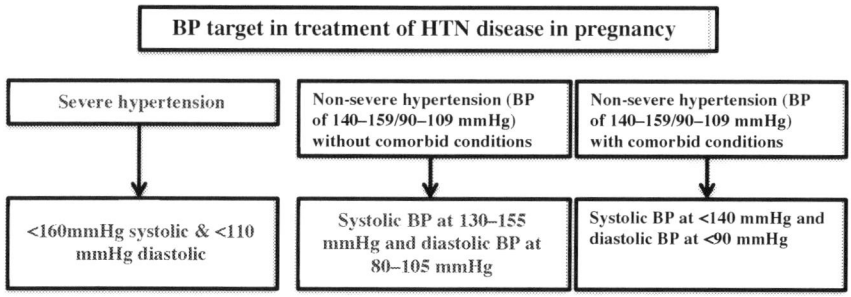

23.6 Time of delivery in chronic HTN patient

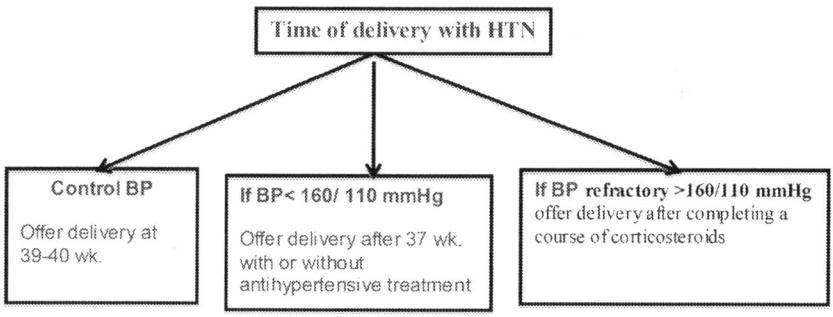

23.7 Post partum follow up with chronic HTN

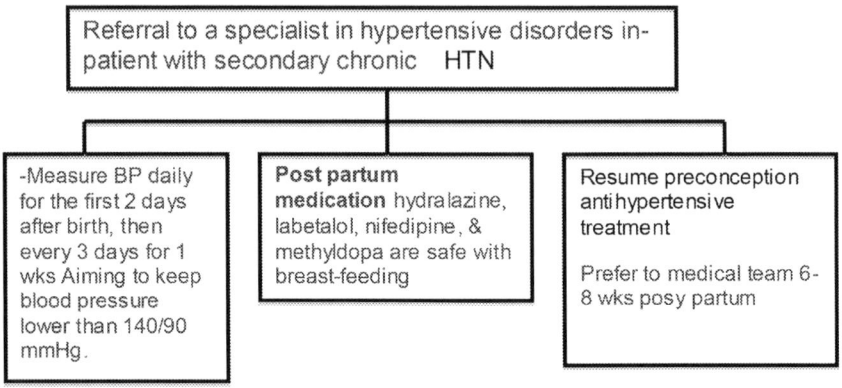

23.8 Gestational hypertension classification

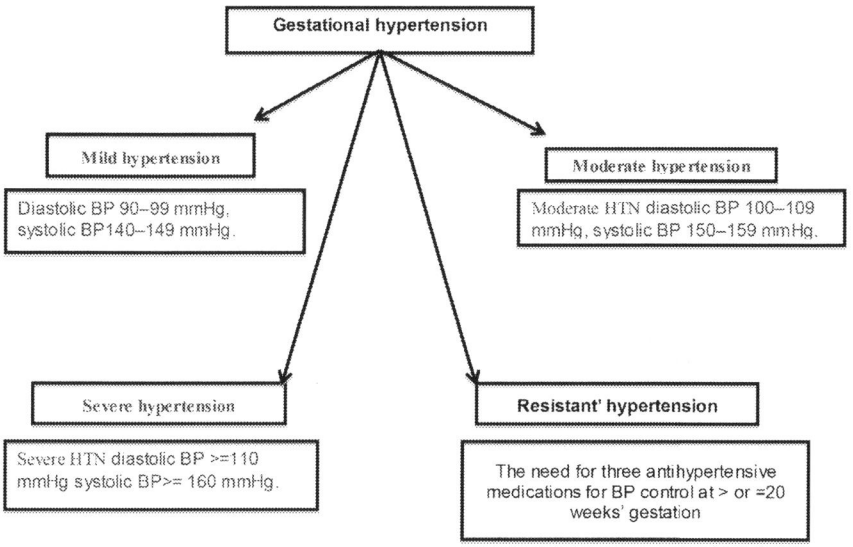

23.9 Gestational hypertension

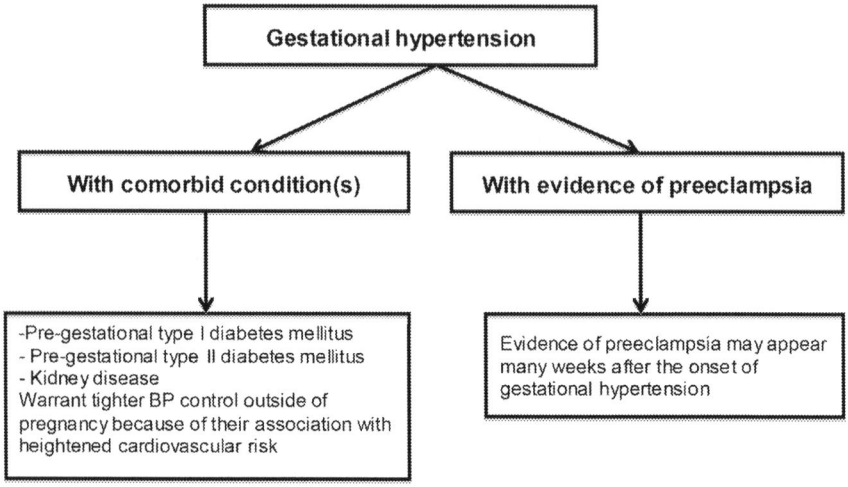

23.10 Management of pregnancy with gestational HTN

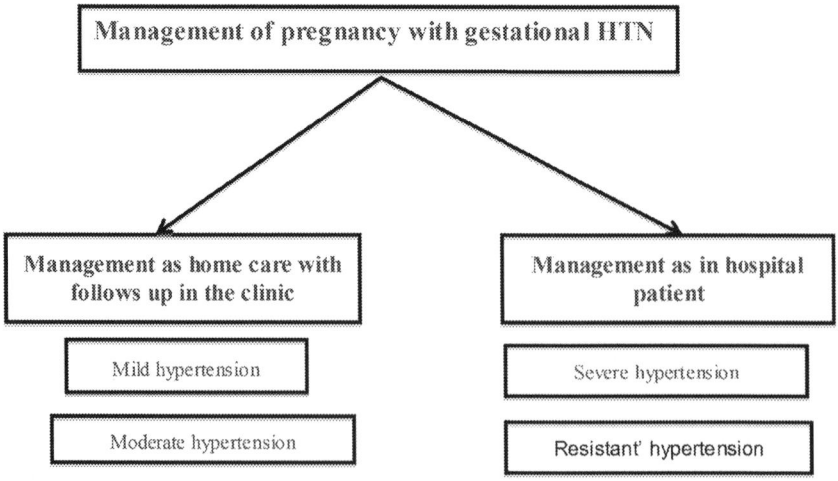

23.11 Preconception advice

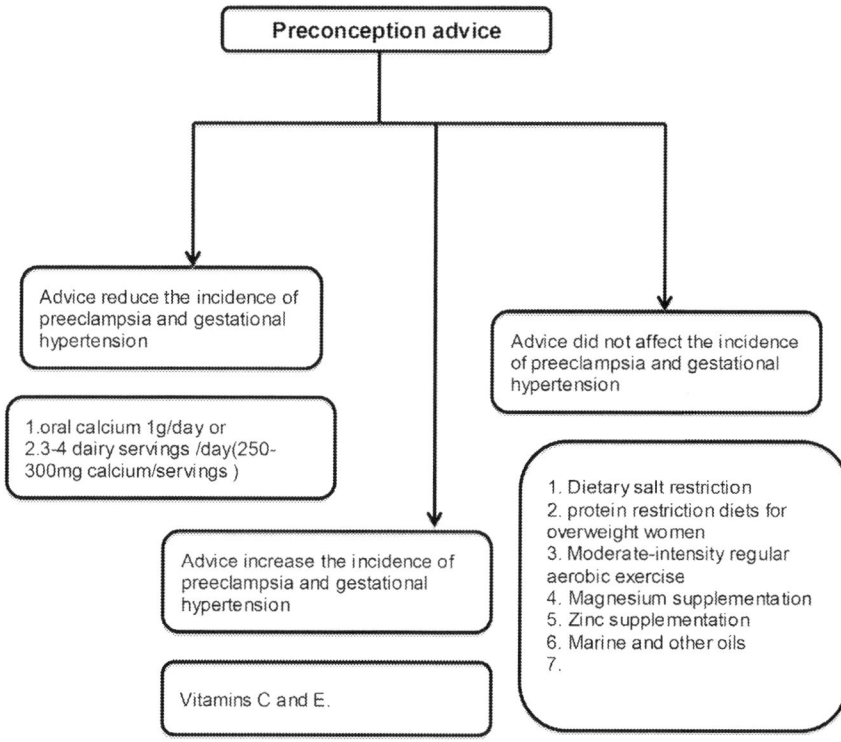

23.12 ANC follow up of patient with gestational hypertension

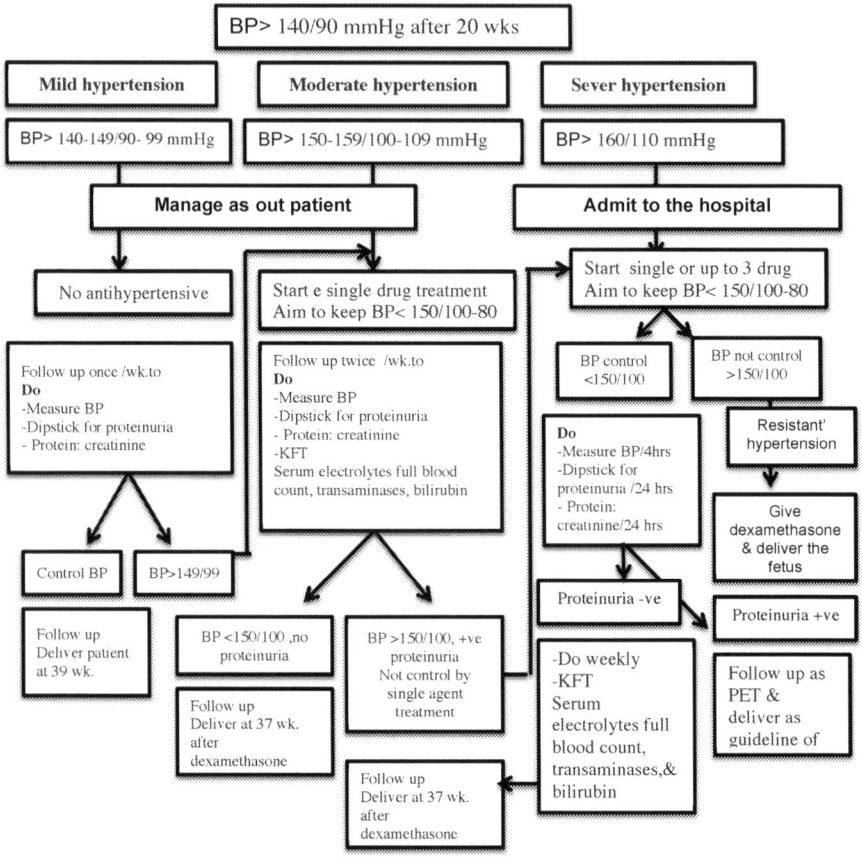

23.13 Time of delivery

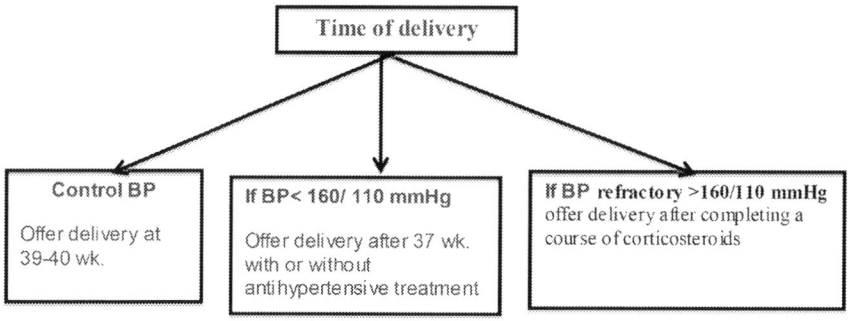

23.14 Postnatal investigation, monitoring and treatment

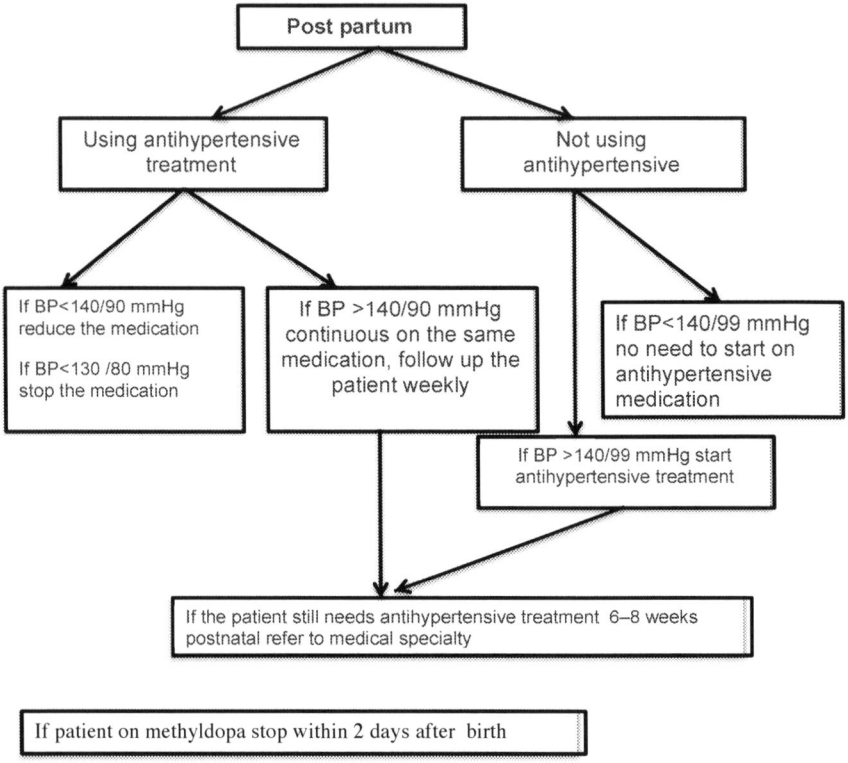

24 Protein S deficiency

Protein S deficiency

Hereditary

- Autosomal dominant trait. Thrombosis is observed in both heterozygous (2% incompatible with life) and homozygous genetic deficiencies of protein S.

-Protein S and C levels are lower in sickle cell anemia and they decrease further significantly during crisis

Acquired

Is usually due to

- Hepatic diseases
- vitamin K deficiency
- result of antagonism with oral warfarin anticoagulants
- low levels of protein S in pregnancy do not cause thrombosis by themselves.
- Disseminated intravascular coagulation
- HIV infection
- The nephrotic syndrome
- Age affects total protein S but not free protein S levels
- Patient recover from chickenpox

24.1 Management of protein S deficiency

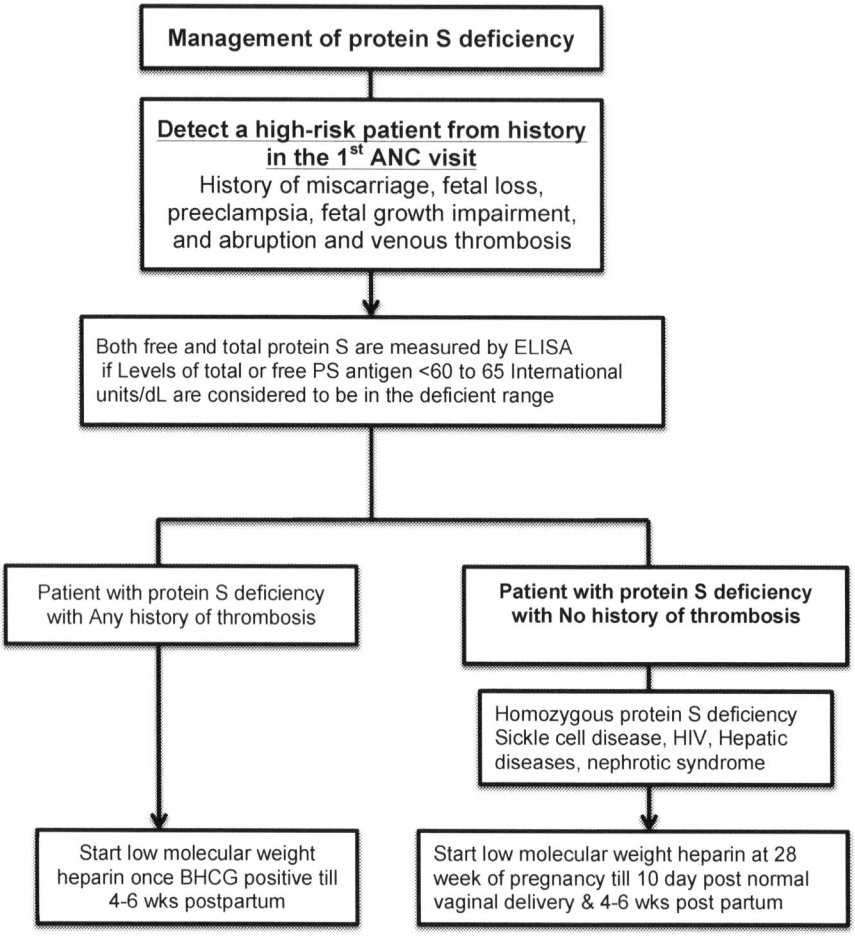

25 Systemic lupus erythematosus

25.1 Clinical course of SLE in pregnancy

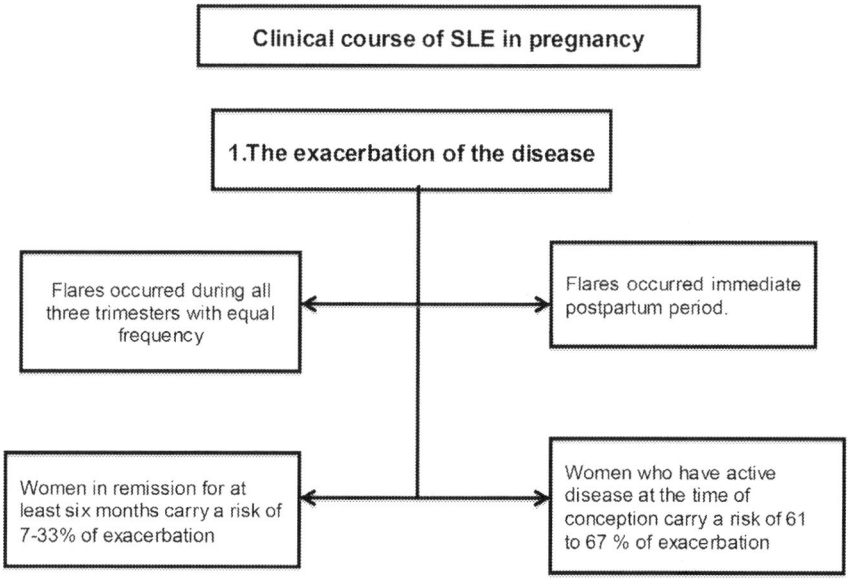

25.2 The exacerbation of renal disease in SLE patient

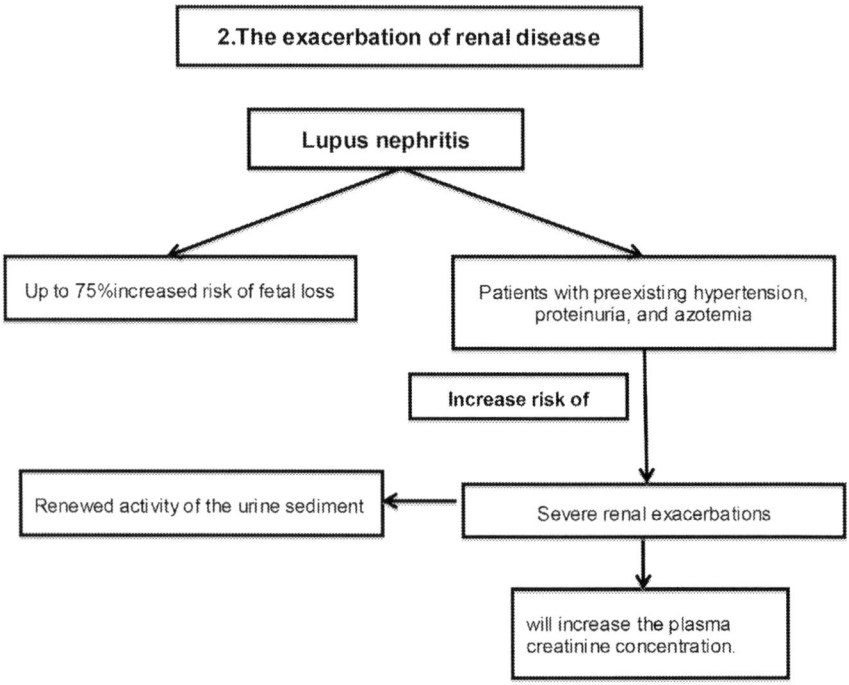

25.3 Pregnancy following renal transplantation

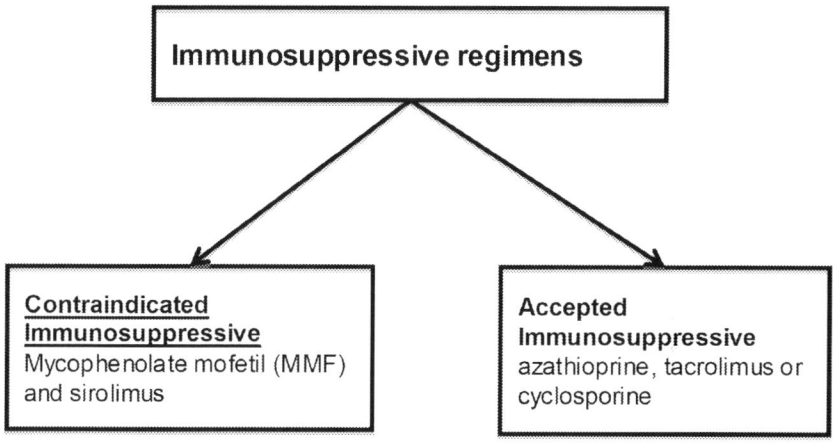

25.4 Treatment of patient with SLE Recommendation

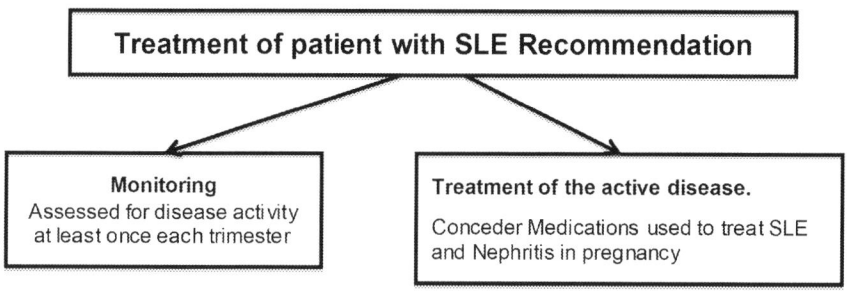

25.5 ANC follow up for patient with SLE

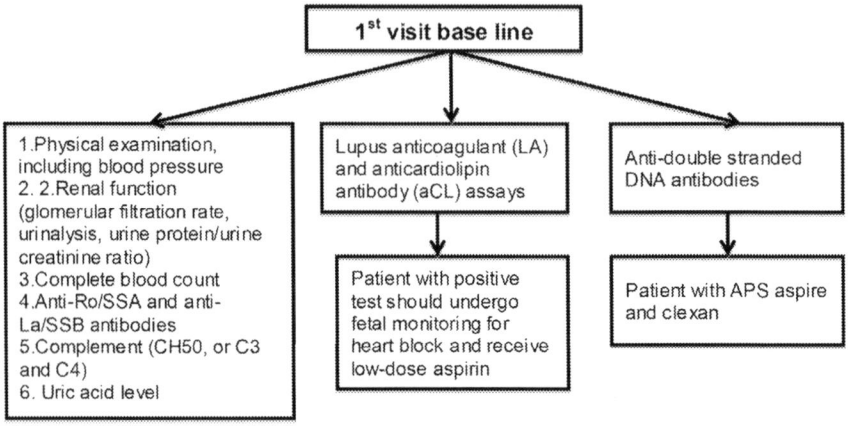

25.6 Monitoring of SLE patient in the last trimester

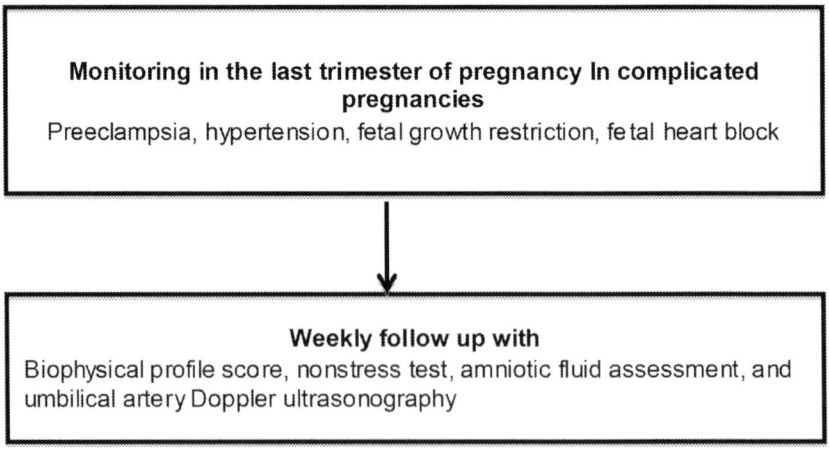

25.7 Management of patient with SLE in the postpartum period

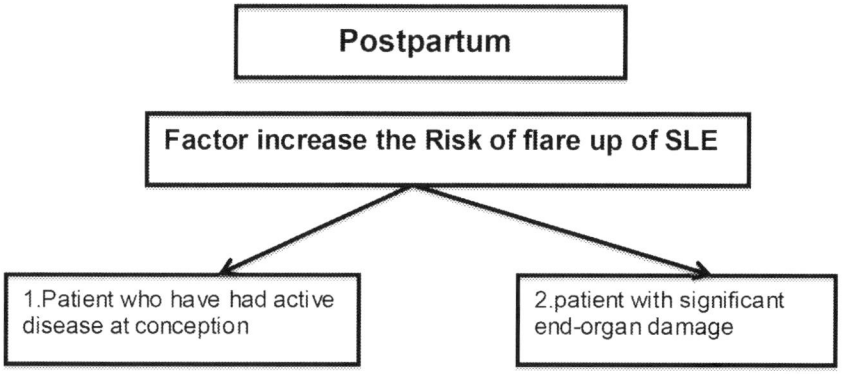

25.8 Drug safe for the nursing infant

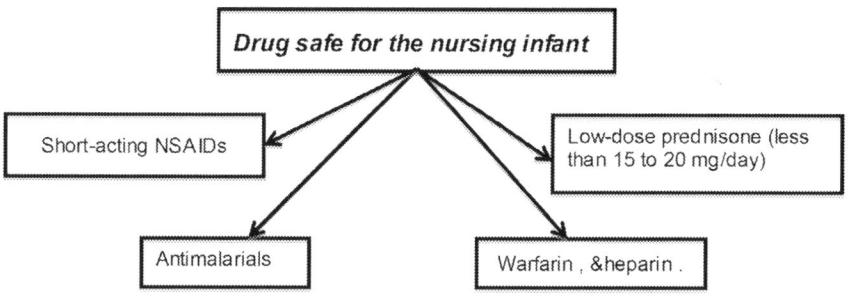

25.9 Treatment of active disease.

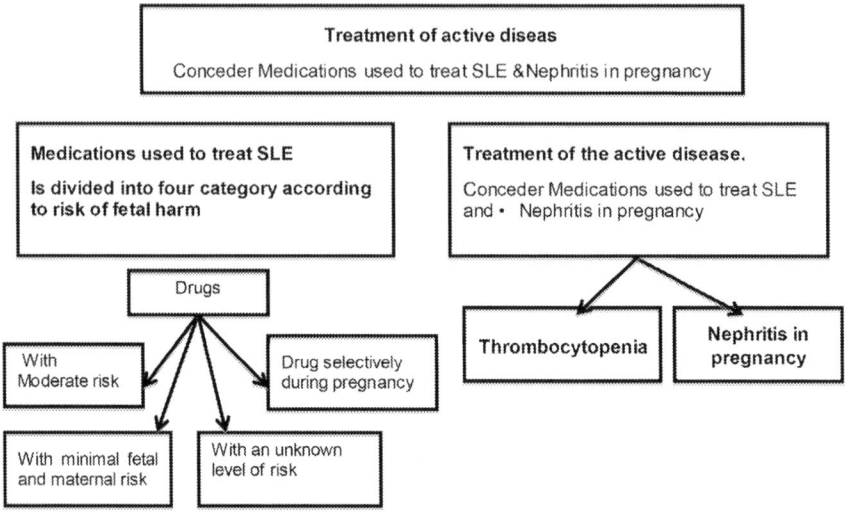

25.10 Drug with Moderate to high risk of fetal harm

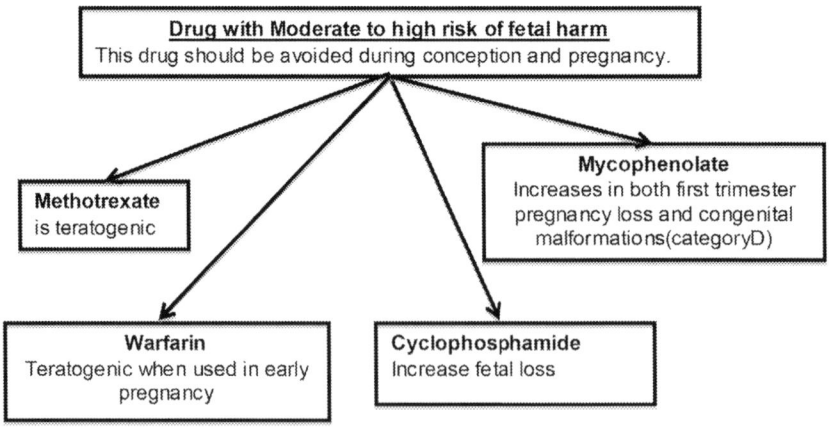

25.11 Drug with Minimal fetal and maternal risk

Drug with Minimal fetal and maternal risk

NSAID use during early and late pregnancy and antimalarial drug use throughout pregnancy are probably safe.

NSAIDs

NSAIDs are safe during the latter part of the first and during the second trimester but should be discontinued in the last trimester of pregnancy.

Antimalarial drugs

The safety of drugs is uncertain, Patients who discontinue hydroxychloroquine prior to, or during, pregnancy are more likely to have exacerbations of SLE

Unknown level of risk

Use of biologic antirheumatic drugs such as B cell targeted antibodies (e.g., rituximab) and T-B cell costimulation blockers (e.g. abatacept) is discouraged in part because of a lack of data on safety of their use during pregnancy.

25.12 Drug with Selective use allowed during pregnancy

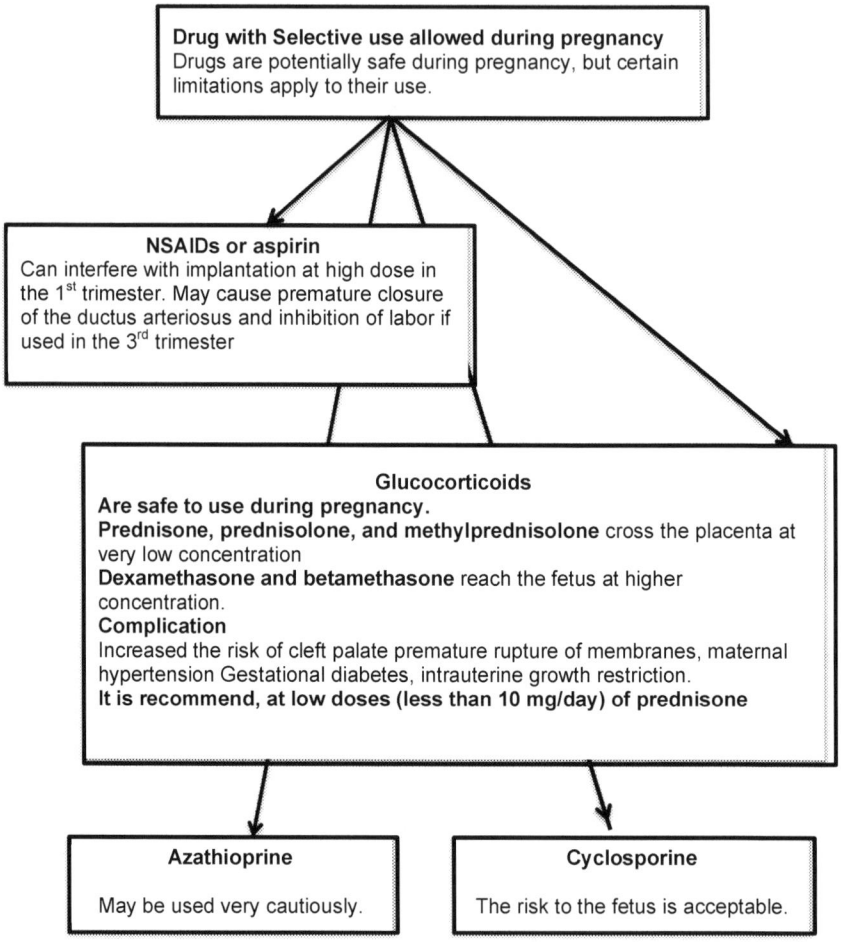

25.13 Thrombocytopenia in SLE

Thrombocytopenia

During lupus pregnancies may have multiple causes

Thrombocytopenia can be due to Antiplatelet antibodies, toxemia, and antiphospholipid antibodies. Treatment includes high-dose prednisone and intravenous immune globulin

26 Pregnancy with kidney disease

26.1 Preconception advice for effect of pregnancy on kidney disease

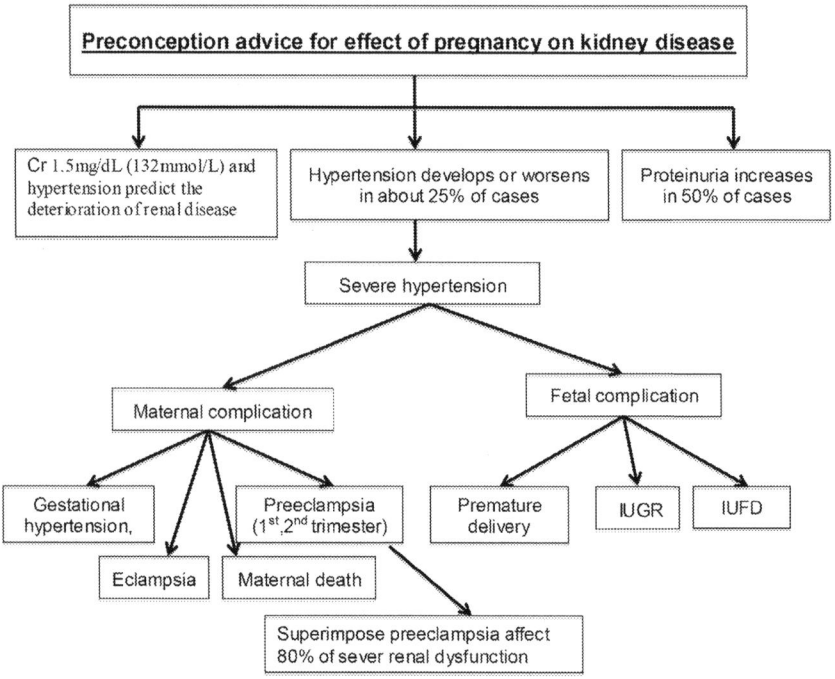

26.2 Effect of pregnancy on renal function RF

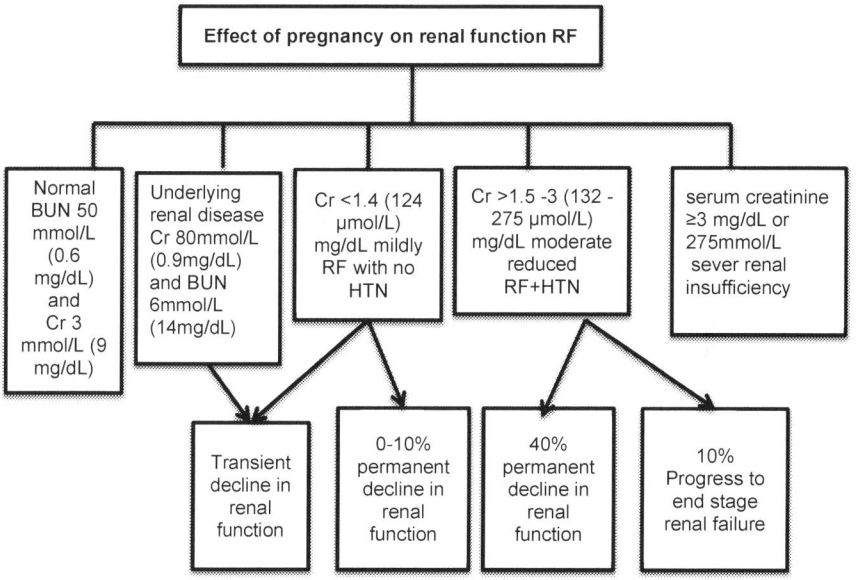

26.3 Management of pregnant women with renal disease

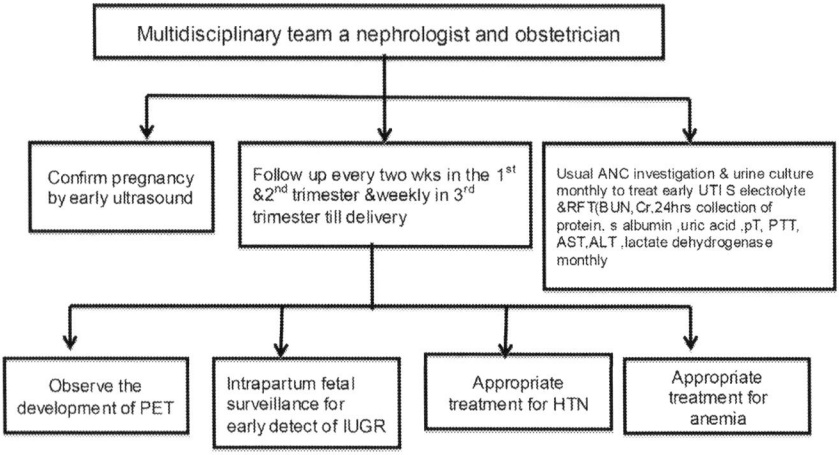

26.4 Special situation in pregnancy with renal disease

Patient with renal transplant

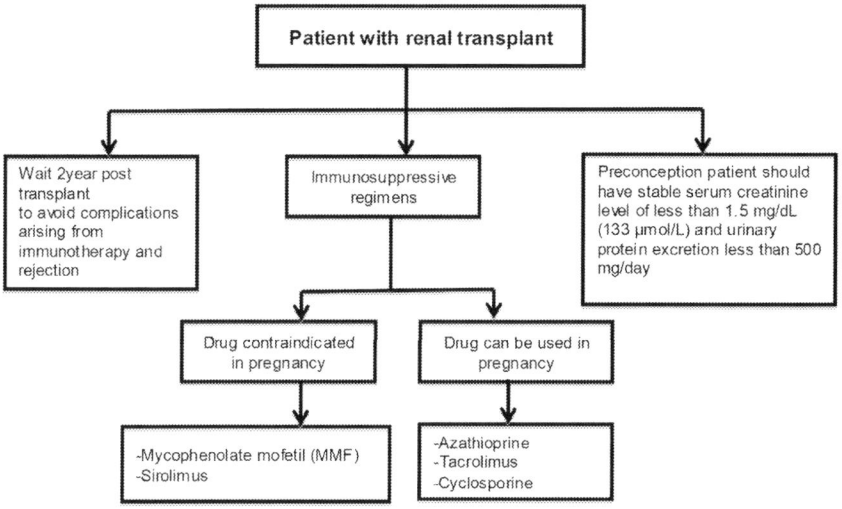

Patient with Intensive dialysis

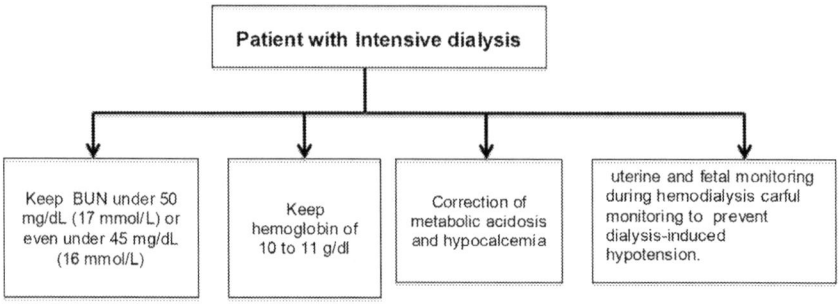

27 Rh and other blood group alloimmunizations

27.1 Follow up of Rh-negative blood group

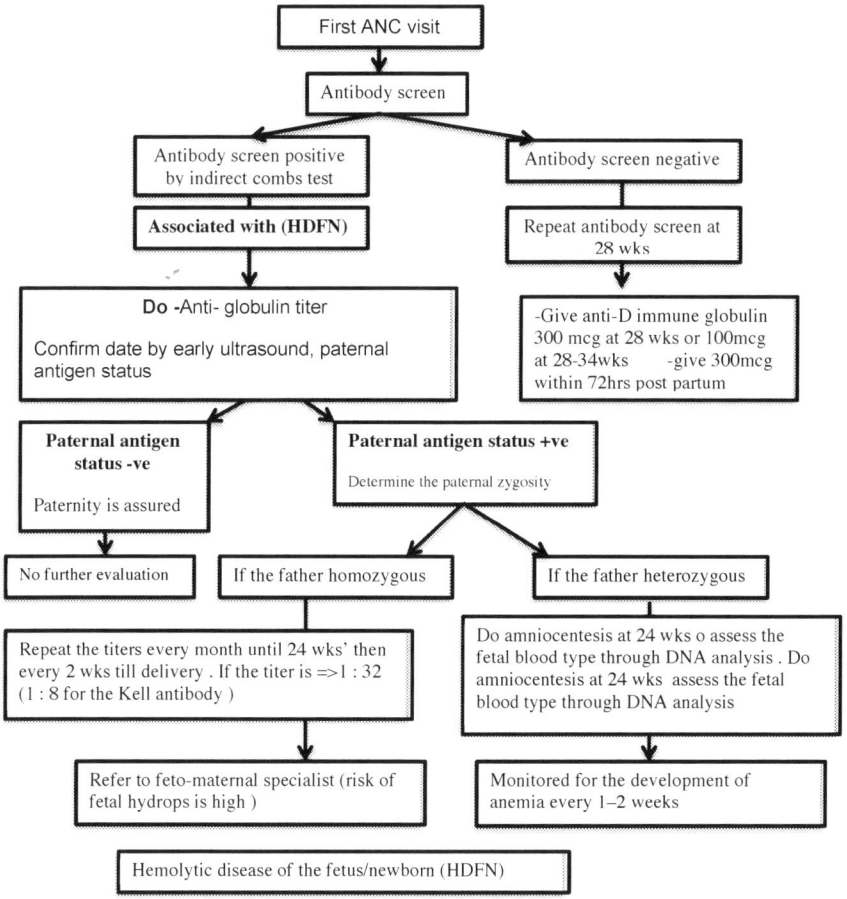

27.2 ANC follow up and Monitored for the development of fetal anemia

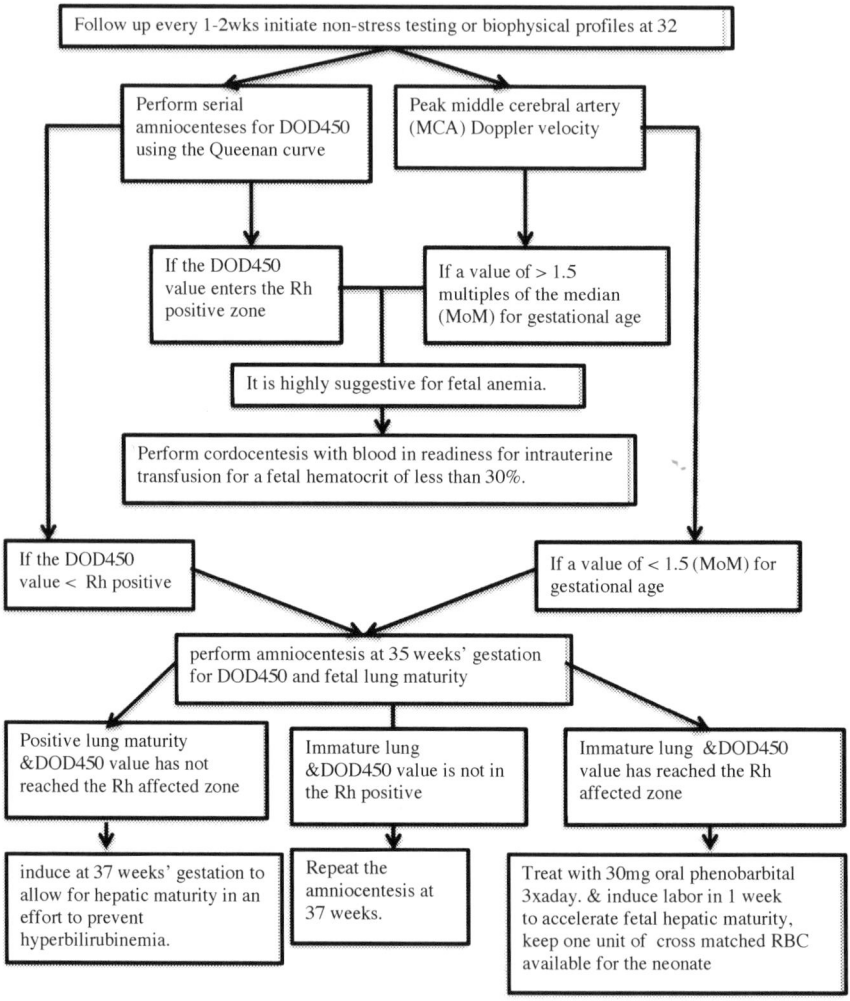

27.3 Management of subsequent Alloimmune pregnancy

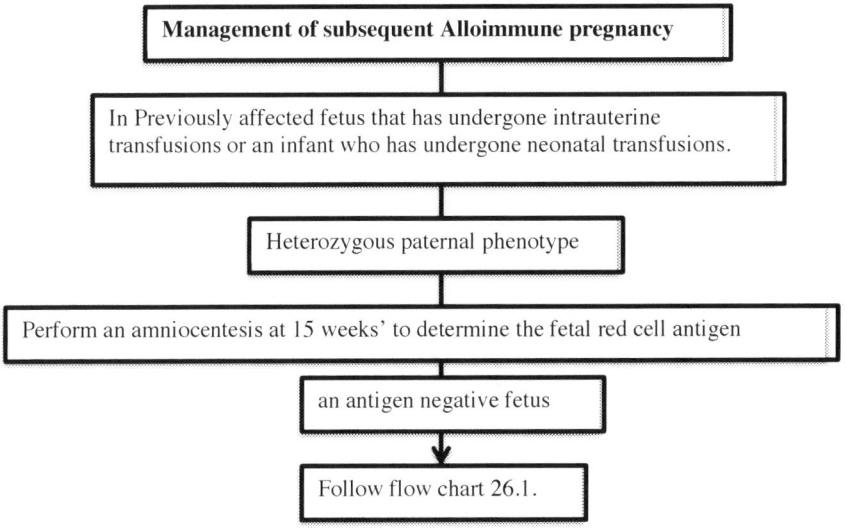

28. Epilepsy in pregnancy

28.1 Preconception advice

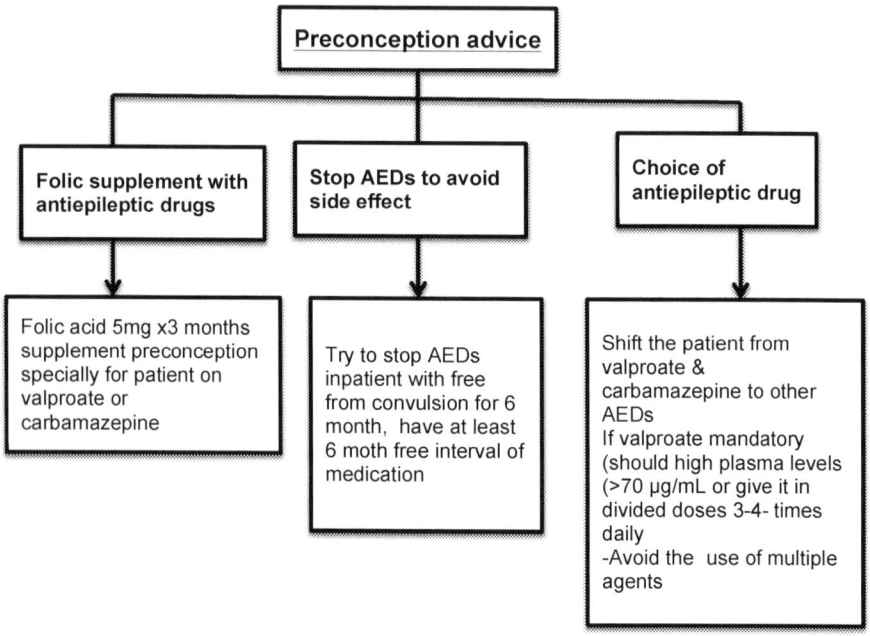

28.2 Management of epileptic patient during pregnancy

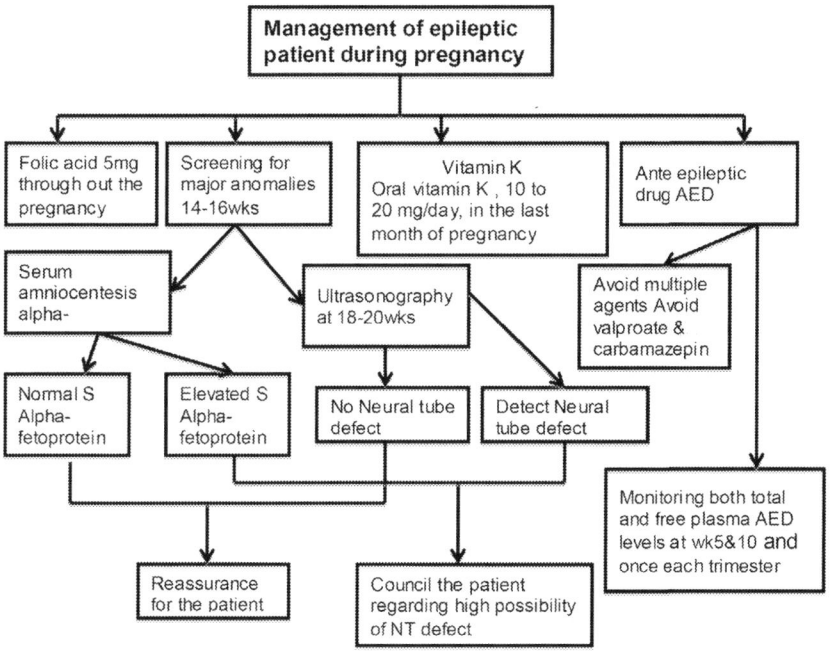

28.3 Mode of delivery in patient with epilepsy

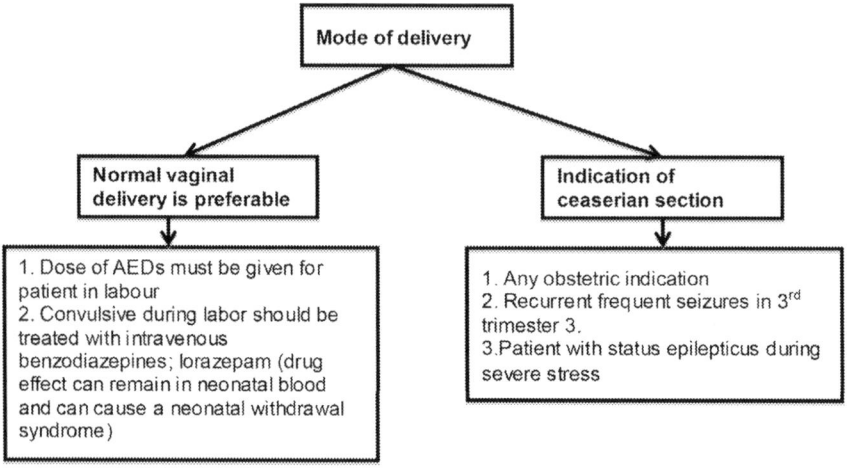

28.4 Post partum care for patient with epilepsy

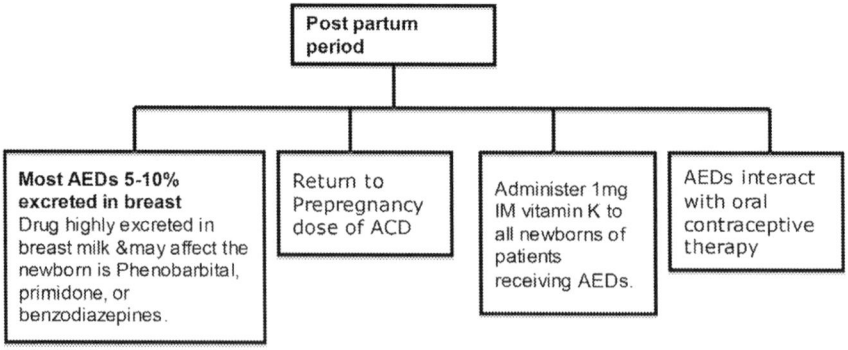

29 Cardiac disease in pregnancy

29.1 type of cardiac diseas in pregnancy

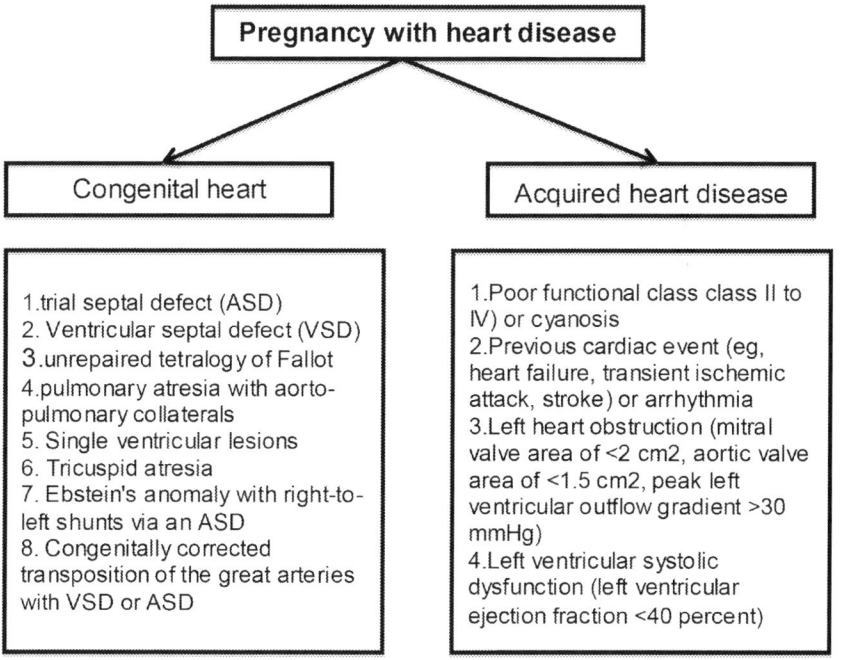

29.2 Condition associated with maternal and fetal risk

Condition associated with maternal and fetal risk

High maternal and fetal risk

1. Severe aortic stenosis with or without symptoms
2.Symptomatic mitral stenosis (NYHA class II to IV)
3.Aortic or mitral regurgitation with NYHA class III to IV symptoms
4.Aortic and/or mitral valve disease with severe left ventricular dysfunction (LVEF < 40 %) or severe pulmonary hypertension (pulmonary artery pressure >75 %of systemic pressure)
5.Marfan syndrome with or without aortic regurgitation
6.Mechanical prosthetic valve requiring anticoagulation

Low maternal and fetal risk

1.Asymptomatic aortic stenosis with an LVEF >50 percent and a mean gradient < 25 mmHg
2.Aortic or mitral regurgitation with no or mild symptoms (NYHA class I to II)
3.Mitral valve prolapse with either no mitral regurgitation or mild to moderate mitral regurgitation with an LVEF >50 percent
4.Mild mitral stenosis (defined as a mitral valve area >1.5 cm2 and a mean gradient less the 5 mmHg) without severe pulmonary hypertension (pulmonary artery pressure >75 percent of systemic pressure)
5.Mild to moderate pulmonary valve stenosis

Cardiac surgery should be avoided during pregnancy due to high risk on the fetus for the fetus, no difference in the maternal risk .

29.3 ANC for patient with cardiac disease

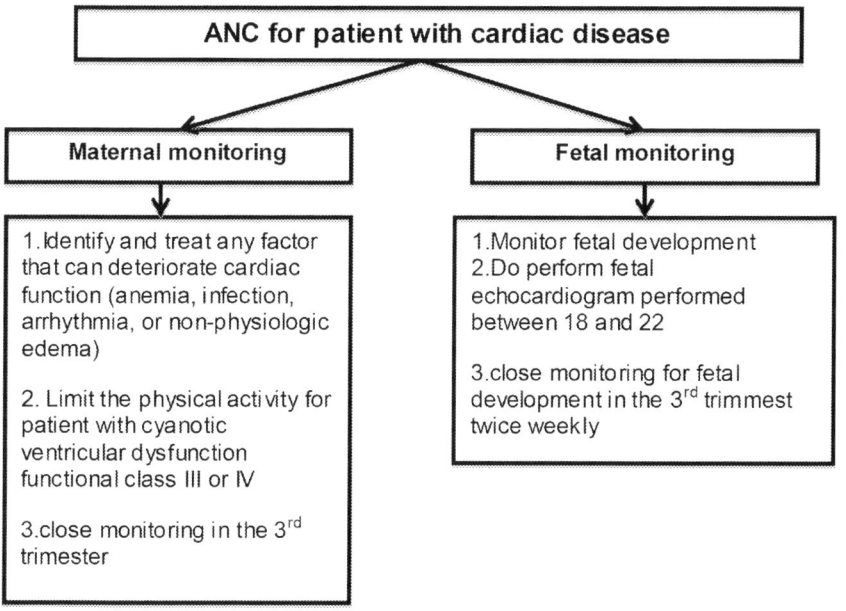

29.4 Mode of delivery in cardiac patient

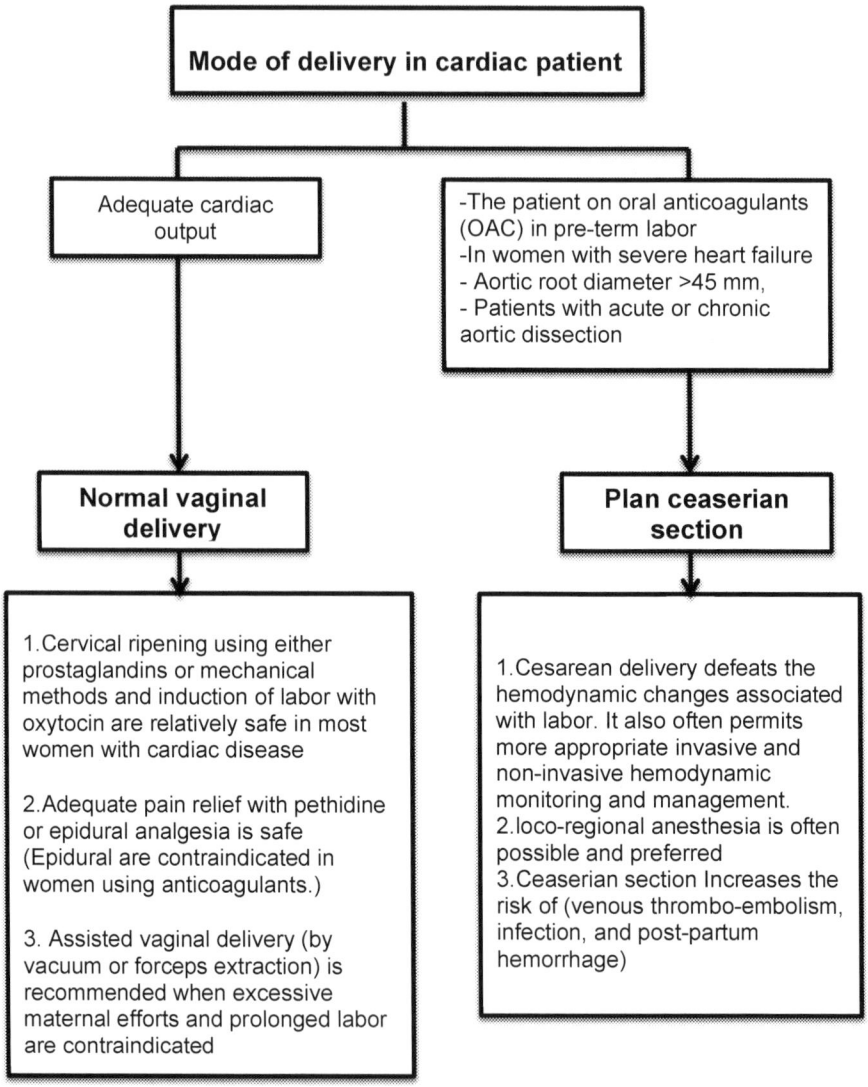

Section II Instruction manual in Labour room

30 Diagnoses and Management of patient in Labor

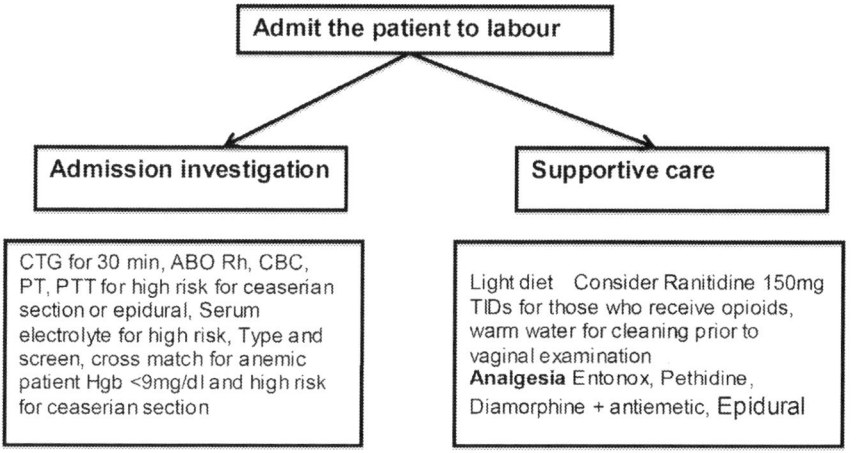

30.1 Patient assessment in emergency room

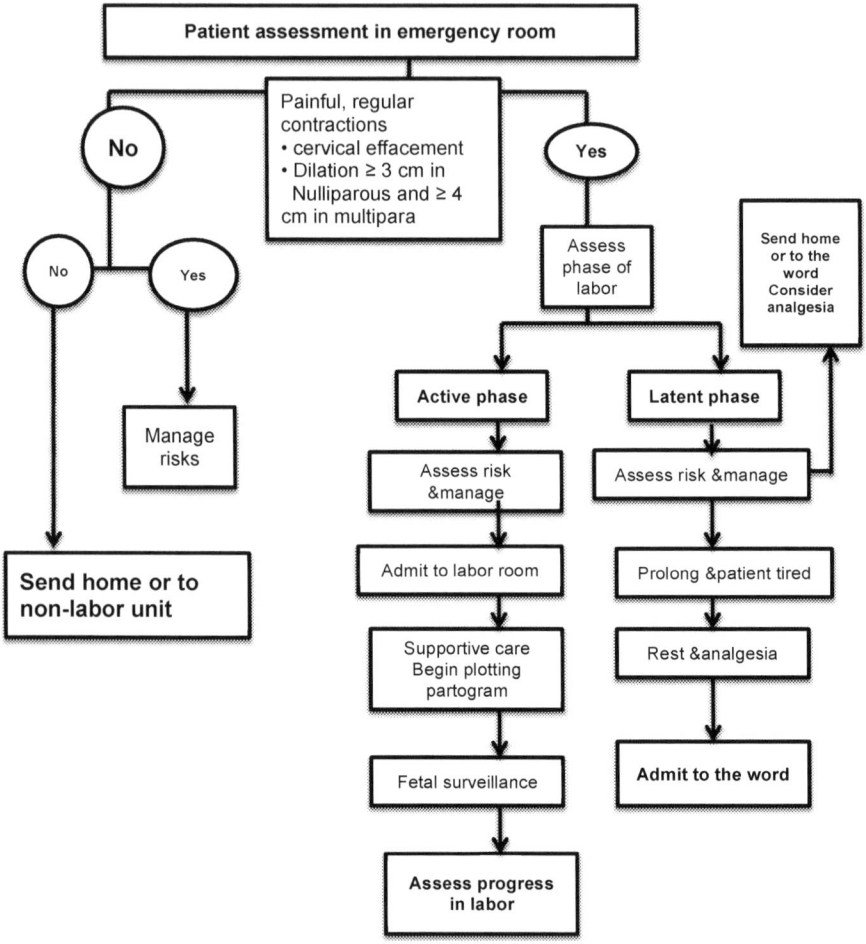

30.2 Patient assessment in labor room

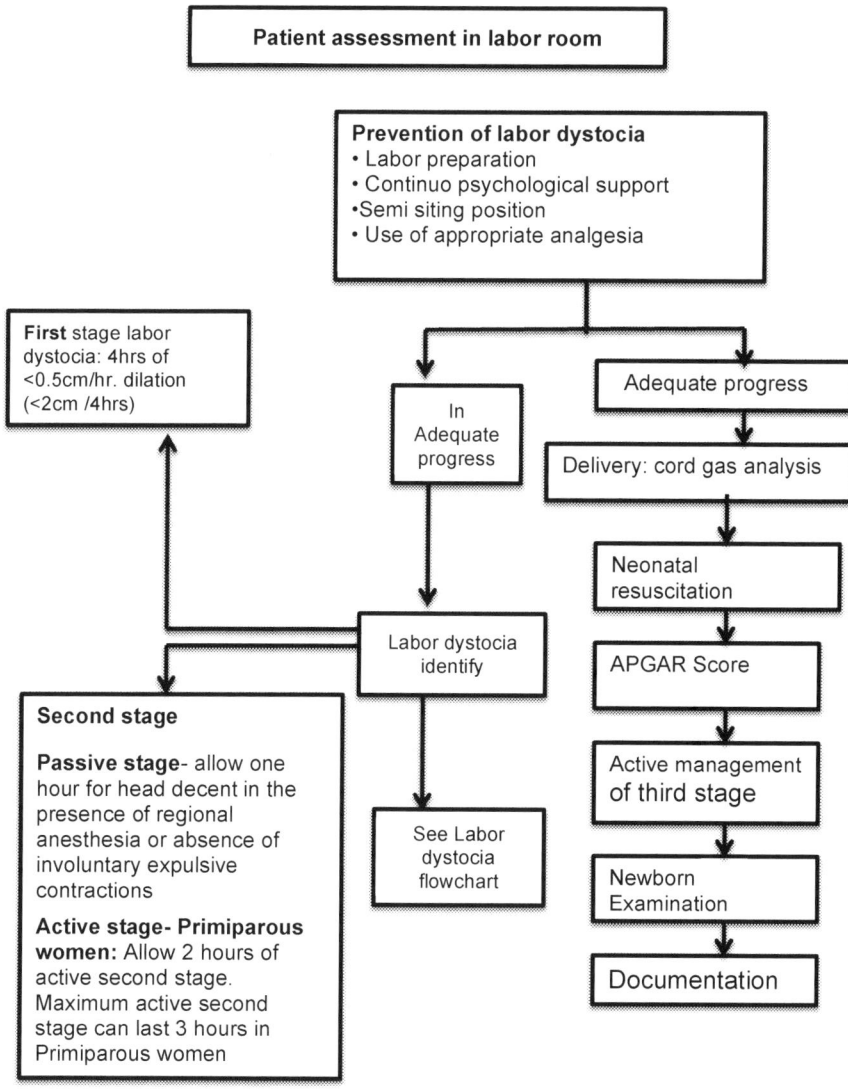

30.3 Third Stage of Labor

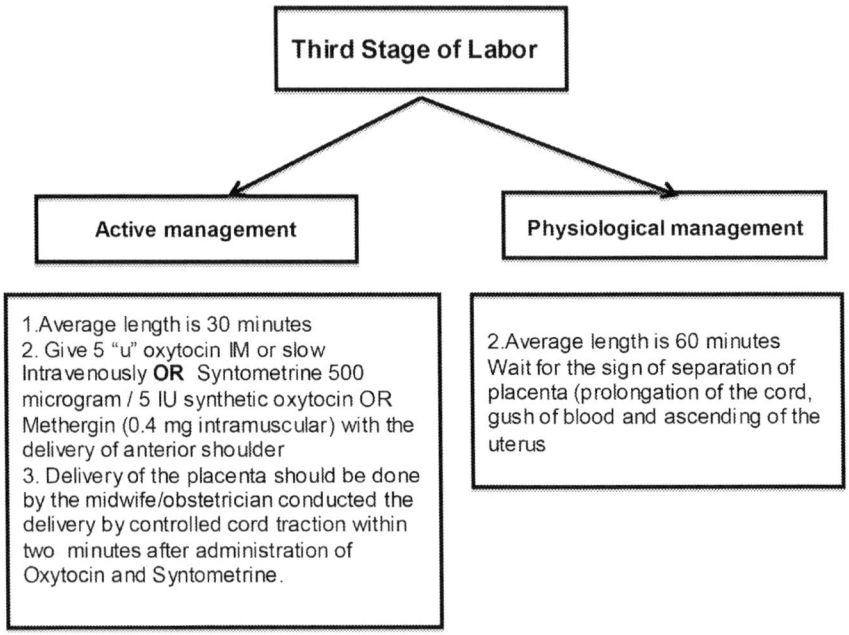

30.4 Category of the CTG

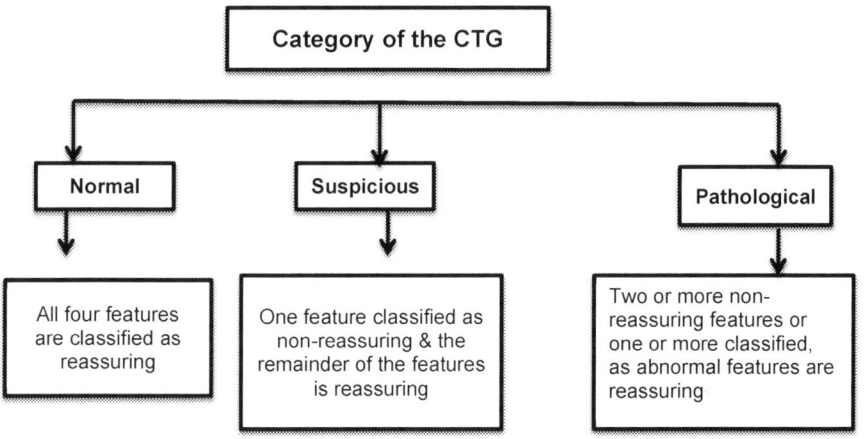

Essential practical point for Performing Electronic Fetal Monitoring (EFM))

- The date and time on the EFM machine should be correctly set, ensure machine is set to 1cm/hour.
- The cardiotocograph label should be used to record mother's name, date of birth and hospital number, maternal pulse rate, reason for EFM, date and time of trace commenced, signature of midwife.
- Any antenatal/intrapartum events that may affect the FH rate should be noted contemporaneously on the CTG and in the maternal notes, signed and the date and time noted (VE's, FBS sampling, siting of an epidural)•

30.5 Categorization of Fetal Heart Rate

Feature	Baseline (b/pm)	Variability (b/pm)	Decelerations
Reassuring	110-160	>5	None
Non-reassuring	161–180	Less than 5 for 30–90 minutes	Variable decelerations: Dropping from baseline by 60 beats/ minute or less and taking 60 seconds or less to recover Present for over 90 minutes Occurring with over 50% of contractions. **OR** Variable decelerations: Dropping from baseline by more than 60 beats/ minute or taking over 60 seconds to recover present for up to 30 minutes occurring with over 50% of contractions. **OR** Late decelerations: present for up to 30 minutes Occurring with over 50% of contractions

Abnormal	Above 180 Or below 100	Less than 5 for over 90 minutes	Non-reassuring variable decelerations (see row above): still observed 30 minutes after starting conservative measures occurring with over 50% of contractions. OR Late decelerations: present for over 30 minutes Do not improve with conservative measures Occurring with over 50% of contractions. OR Bradycardia or a single prolonged deceleration lasting 3 minutes or more.

30.6 Management of CTG:

Category	Definition	Interpretation	Management
CTG is normal/ reassuring	All 3 features are normal/ reassuring	Normal CTG, no non-reassuring or abnormal features, healthy fetus	Continue CTG and normal care. If CTG was started because of concerns Arising from intermittent auscultation, Remove CTG after 20 minutes if there are no non-reassuring or abnormal features and no ongoing risk factors.

CTG is non-reassuring and suggests need for conservative measures	1 non-reassuring feature AND 2 normal/ reassuring features	Combination of features that may be associated with increased risk of fetal acidosis; if accelerations are present, acidosis is unlikely	Think about possible underlying causes. If the baseline fetal heart rate is over 160 beats/ minute, Check the woman's temperature and pulse. If either are raised, offer fluids & paracetamol. Start 1 or more conservative measures: Encourage the woman to mobilise or adopt a left-lateral position,& in particular To avoid being supine offer oral or intravenous fluids reduce contraction frequency by stopping oxytocin if being used and/or offering tocolysis. Inform coordinating midwife & obstetrician.

CTG is abnormal and indicates need for conservative measures AND further testing	1 abnormal feature OR 2 non-reassuring features	Combination of features that is more likely to be associated with fetal acidosis	CTG is abnormal and indicates need for conservative Measures AND further testing 1 abnormal feature OR 2 non-reassuring features Combination of features that is more likely to be associated with fetal acidosis Discuss with the consultant obstetrician if an FBS cannot be obtained or a third FBS is thought to be needed.

CTG is abnormal and indicates need for urgent intervention	Bradycardia or a single prolonged deceleration with baseline below 100 beats/ minute, persisting for 3 minutes or more*	An abnormal feature that is very likely to be associated with current fetal acidosis or imminent rapid development of fetal acidosis	Start 1 or more conservative measures (See 'CTG is non-reassuring...' row for details). Inform coordinating midwife. Urgently seek obstetric help. Make preparations for urgent birth. Expedite birth if persists for 9 minutes. If heart rate recovers before 9 minutes, Reassess decision to expedite birth in discussion With the woman.

Abbreviations: CTG, cardiotocograph; FBS, fetal blood sample.

A stable baseline value of 90–99 beats/minute with normal baseline variability (having confirmed that this is not the maternal heart rate) may be a normal variation; obtain a senior obstetric opinion if uncertain.

The presence of fetal heart rate accelerations is generally a sign that the baby is healthy; the absence of accelerations in an otherwise normal cardiotocograph trace does not indicate

30.7 Classification of Fetal Blood Sample Results

FETAL pH	***SUBSEQUENT ACTION***
>/=7.25	Repeat FBS within 1 hour if the FHR remains pathological
7.21-7.24	Repeat FBS within 30 minutes if the FHR remains pathological or consider Delivery if rapid fall since the last sample
</=7.20	Delivery indicated

31 Regimen for Syntocinon Infusion

Regimen A Primigravida

*10 unit oxytocin in 500 ml 1 mile international Unit =3ml micro drop/min(3ml/hrs)

MiliInternational unit/min	Micro drop/min (mL/hr.)
2	6
4	12
6	18
8	24
10	30
12	36
14	42
16	48
18	54
20	60
22	66
24	72
26	78
28	84
30	90
32	96
34	102
36	108
38	114
40	120

Regimen B Multigravida *10 unit oxytocin in 500 ml 1 mile international Unit =3ml micro drop/min(3ml/hrs)

Mili International unit/min	Micro drop/min (mL/hr.)
1	3
2	6
3	9
4	12
5	15
6	18
7	21
8	24
9	27
10	30
11	33
12	36
13	39
14	42
15	45
16	48
17	51
18	54
19	57
20	60
21	63
22	66
23	69
24	72
25	75
26	78
27	81

28	84
29	87
30	90
31	93
32	96
33	99
34	102
35	105
36	108

Syntocinon should not be started for six hours following administration of vaginal prostaglandins gel and half an hour after Propess.

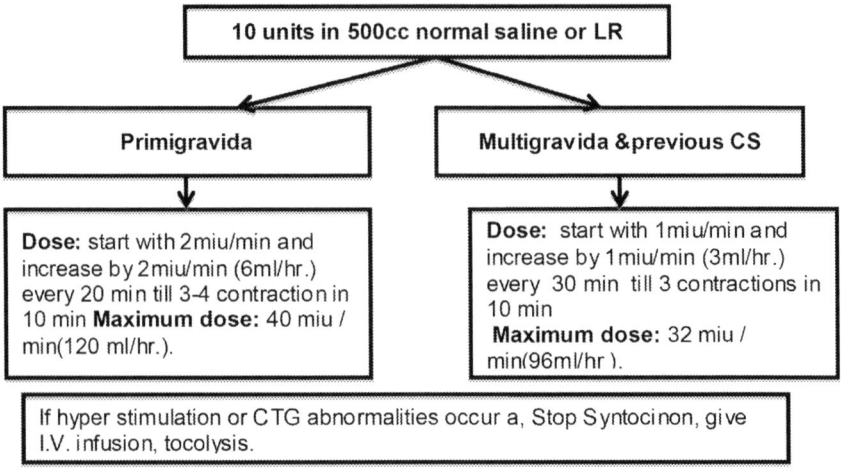
10 units in 500cc normal saline or LR
Primigravida
Multigravida &previous CS
Dose: start with 2miu/min and increase by 2miu/min (6ml/hr.) every 20 min till 3-4 contraction in 10 min Maximum dose: 40 miu / min(120 ml/hr.).
Dose: start with 1miu/min and increase by 1miu/min (3ml/hr.) every 30 min till 3 contractions in 10 min
Maximum dose: 32 miu / min(96ml/hr).
If hyper stimulation or CTG abnormalities occur a, Stop Syntocinon, give I.V. infusion, tocolysis.

32 Cord Blood Sampling

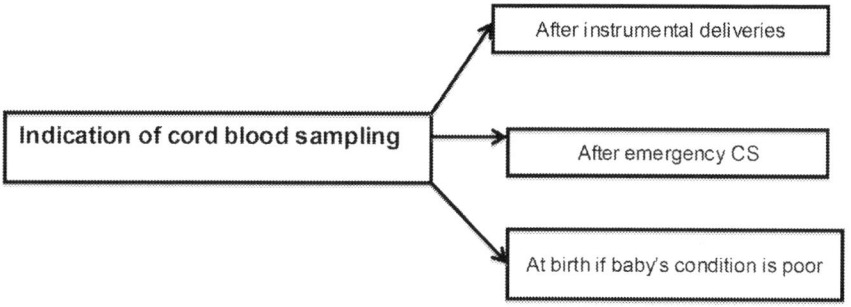

Procedure: Double clamp umbilical cord, collect paired samples from the umbilical artery and umbilical vein either with a pre-heparinized syringe or a pre-heparinized tube. NB: the specimen remains stable at room temperature for up to 1 hour. **Interpretation:** Lower limit of normal may range from 7.02 - 7.18 but the risk of mortality and morbidity does not increase unless the value is < 7.00 and even then the risk is small.

Values of <7.1 should be reported

Cases with ph<7.1 with BD>10 should be audited

33 Guidelines for the care of women' presenting in labor

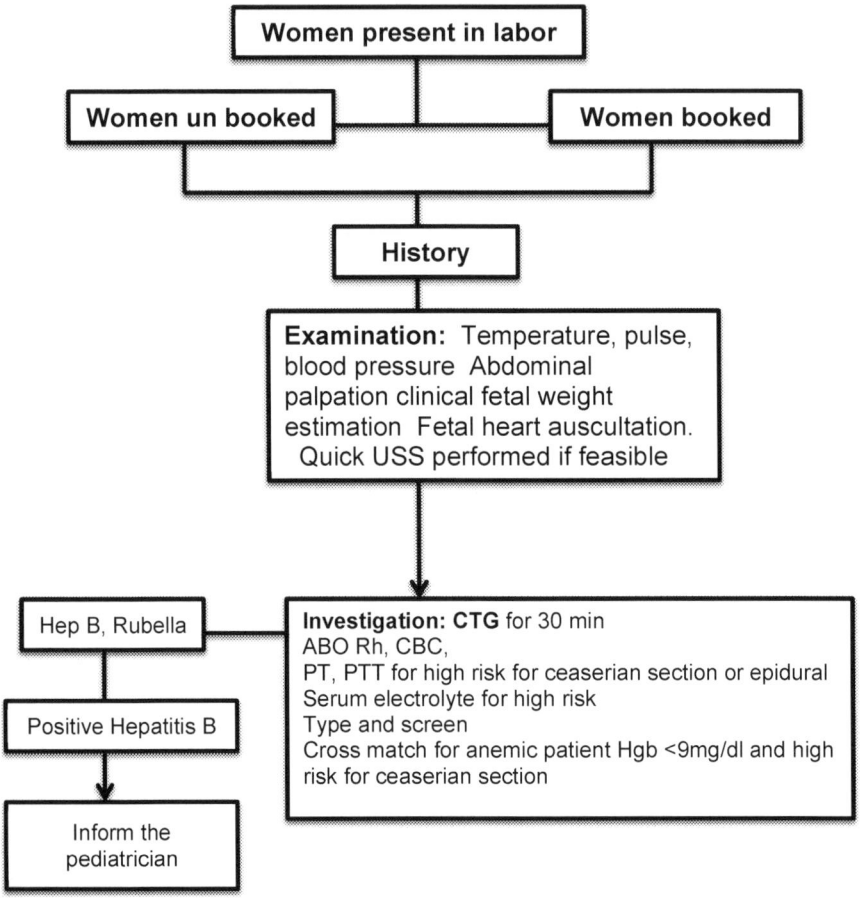

34 Group B Streptococcus (GBS) in Labor

34.1 Prevention of Perinatal Group B Streptococcal (GBS) Disease

Intrapartum antibiotic prophylaxis (IAP) is recommended for:

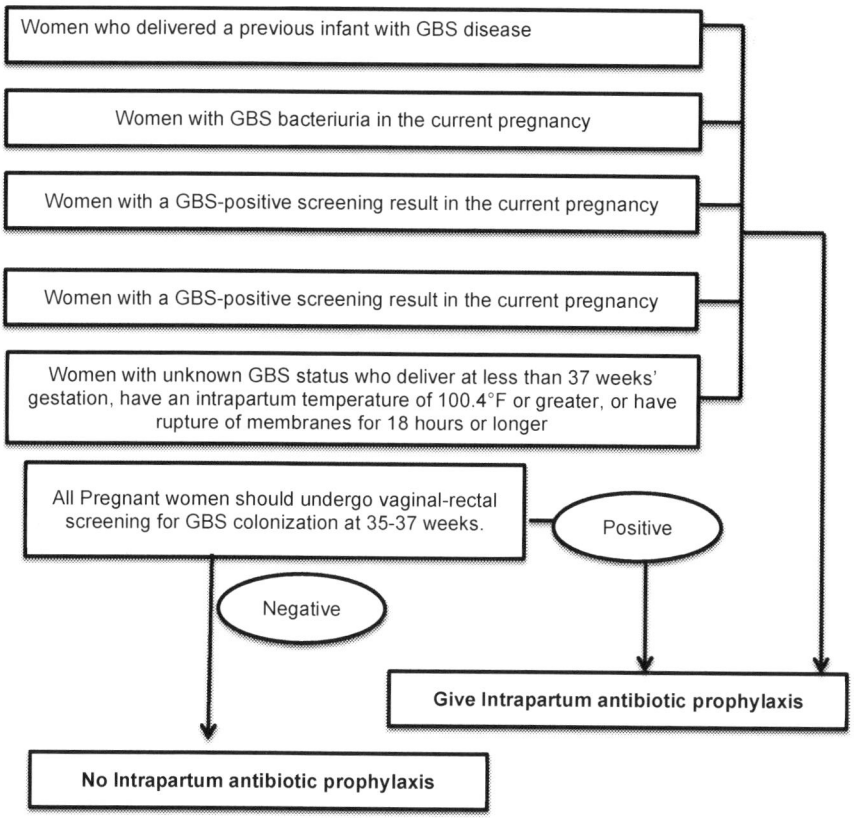

34.2 Recommended regimens for intrapartum antibiotic prophylaxis for prevention of early-onset group B streptococcal (GBS) disease

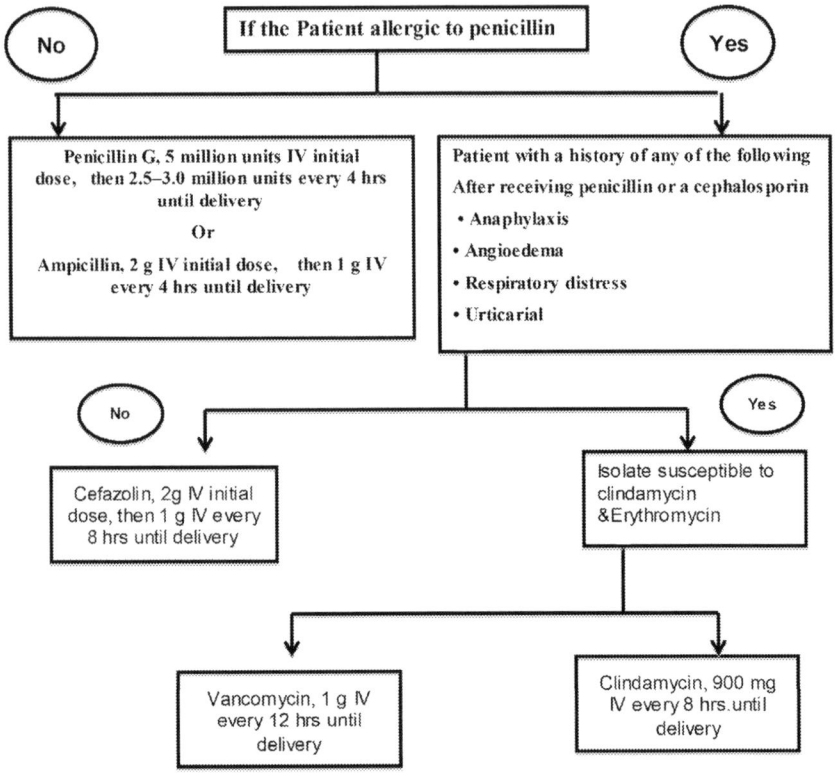

34.3 Group B Streptococcus(GBS) in Labor Pathway

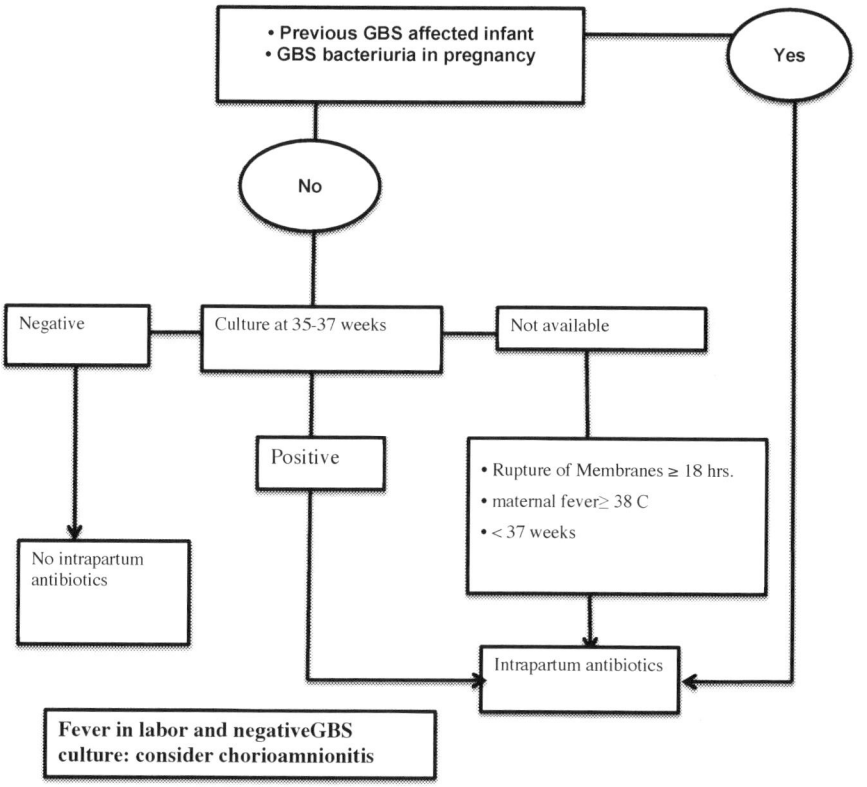

35 Induction of Labor (IOL)

Indication for induction of labor

1.Preeclampsia ≥ 37 weeks

2. Significant maternal disease not responding to treatment

3.Significant but stable antepartum hemorrhage

4.Chorioamnionitis
5.Suspected fetal compromise

6.Term pre-labour rupture of membranes with maternal GBS colonization Postdates (> 41+0 weeks) or post-term (> 42+0 weeks) pregnancy.

Relative indication for induction

-Uncomplicated twin pregnancy ≥ 38 weeks

-Diabetes mellitus (glucose control may dictate urgency)

-Alloimmune disease at or near term

-Intrauterine growth restriction

-Oligohydramnios

-Gestational hypertension ≥ 38 weeks

-Intrauterine fetal death

-PROM at or near term, GBS negative

-Logistical problems (history of rapid labour, distance to hospital)

-Intrauterine death in a prior pregnancy (Induction may be performed to alleviate parental anxiety, but there is no known medical or outcome advantage for mother or baby.

-SLE at 38 wks.

Contraindication

1. Placenta or vasa previa or cord presentation
2. Abnormal fetal lie or presentation (e.g. transverse lie or footling breech)
3. Prior classical or inverted T uterine incision
4. Significant prior uterine surgery (e.g. full thickness myomectomy)
5. Active genital herpes
6. Pelvic structural deformities

Placenta or vasa previa or cord presentation

- Abnormal fetal lie or presentation (e.g. transverse lie or footling breech)
- Prior classical or inverted T uterine incision
- significant prior uterine surgery (e.g. full thickness myomectomy)
- Active genital herpes
- Pelvic structural deformities

Unacceptable indications

1.Care provider or patient convenience

2.Suspected fetal macrosomia (estimated fetal weight > 4000 gm.) in a non-diabetic women is an unacceptable indication because there is no reduction in the incidence of shoulder dystocia but twice the risk of CS.

35.1 Defention needed in induction of labor

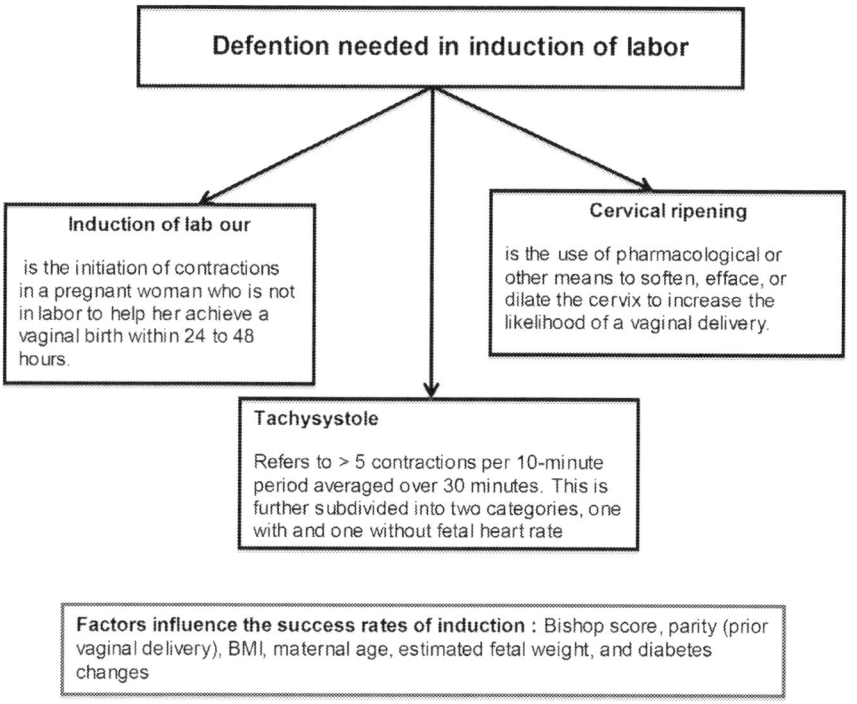

Factors influence the success rates of induction : Bishop score, parity (prior vaginal delivery), BMI, maternal age, estimated fetal weight, and diabetes changes

35.2 Modified Bishop Scoring System

Score

Factor	0	1	2
Dilatation/cm	0	1-2	3-4
Effacement, %	0-30	40-50	60-70
Length, cm	>3	1-3	<1
Consistency	firm	medium	Soft
Position	Posterior	mid	Anterior
Station	Sp-3or above	Sp-2	Sp-1 or0

A favorable pre- induction Bishop score of > 6 are predictive of a successful vaginal delivery.

1. Health care providers should assess the cervix (using the Bishop score) to determine the likelihood of success and to select the appropriate method of induction.

35.3 Ripening / induction: of unfavorable Cervix

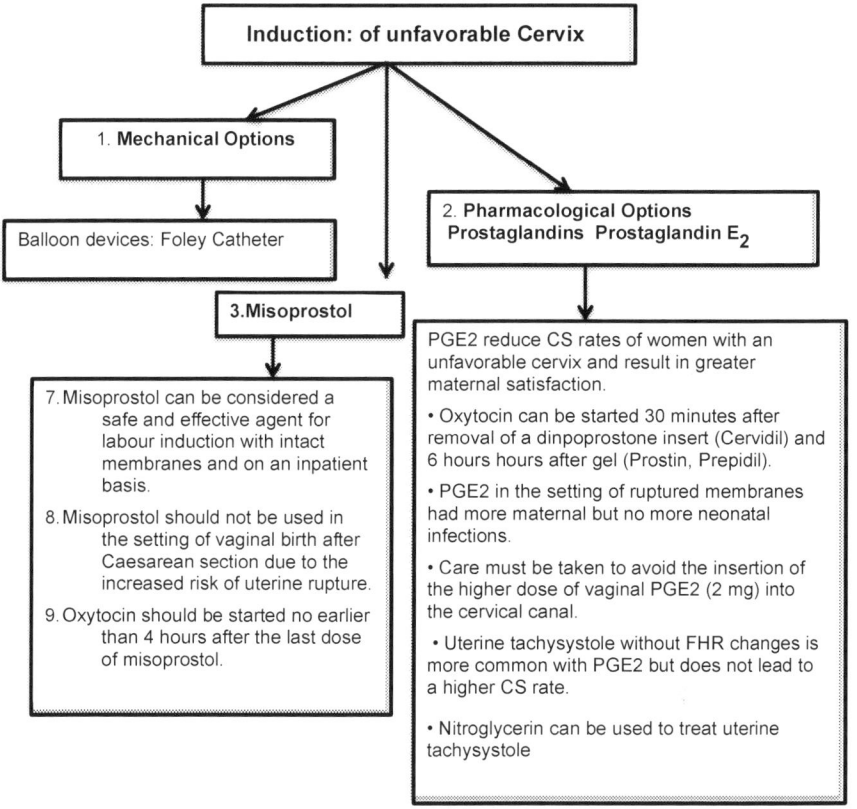

35.4 Induction With a Favorable Cervix

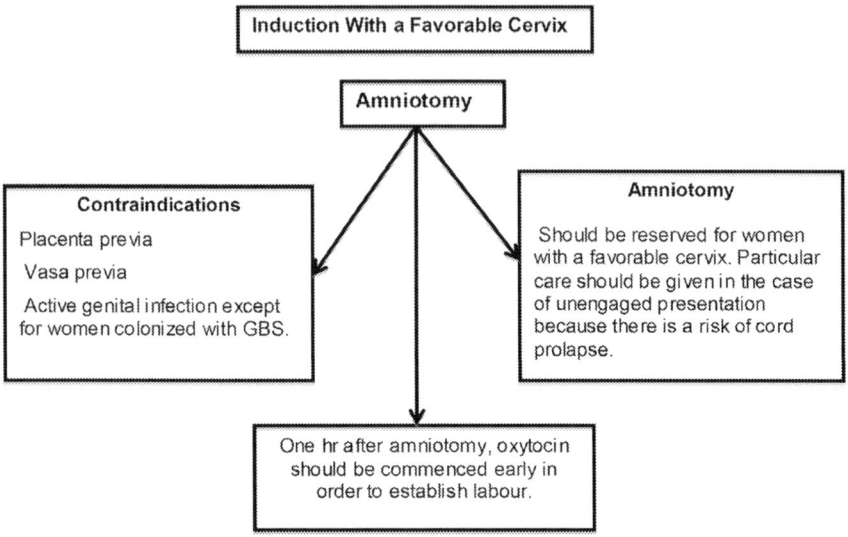

35.5 Induction of labor pathway

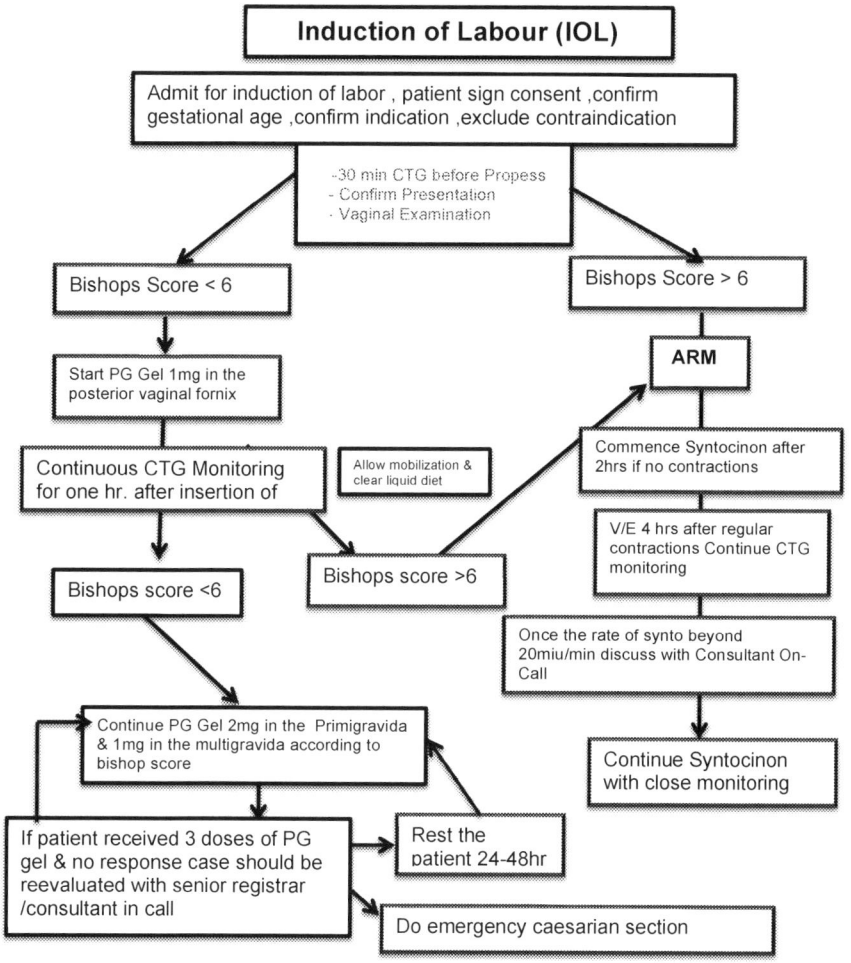

36 The Management of Third- and Fourth-Degree Perineal Tears

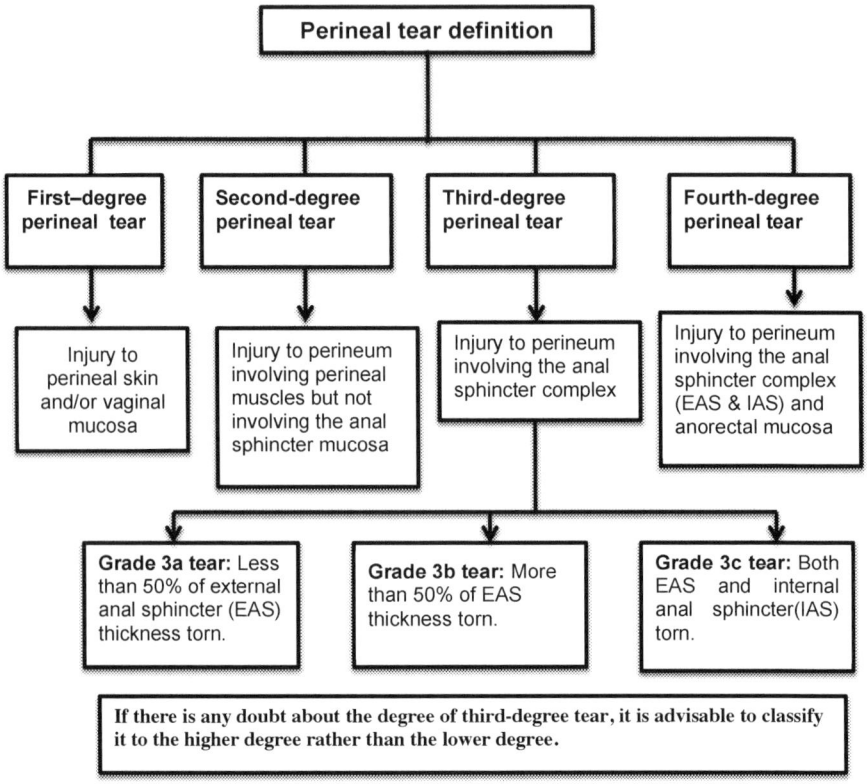

36.1 Repair of third- and fourth-degree pathway

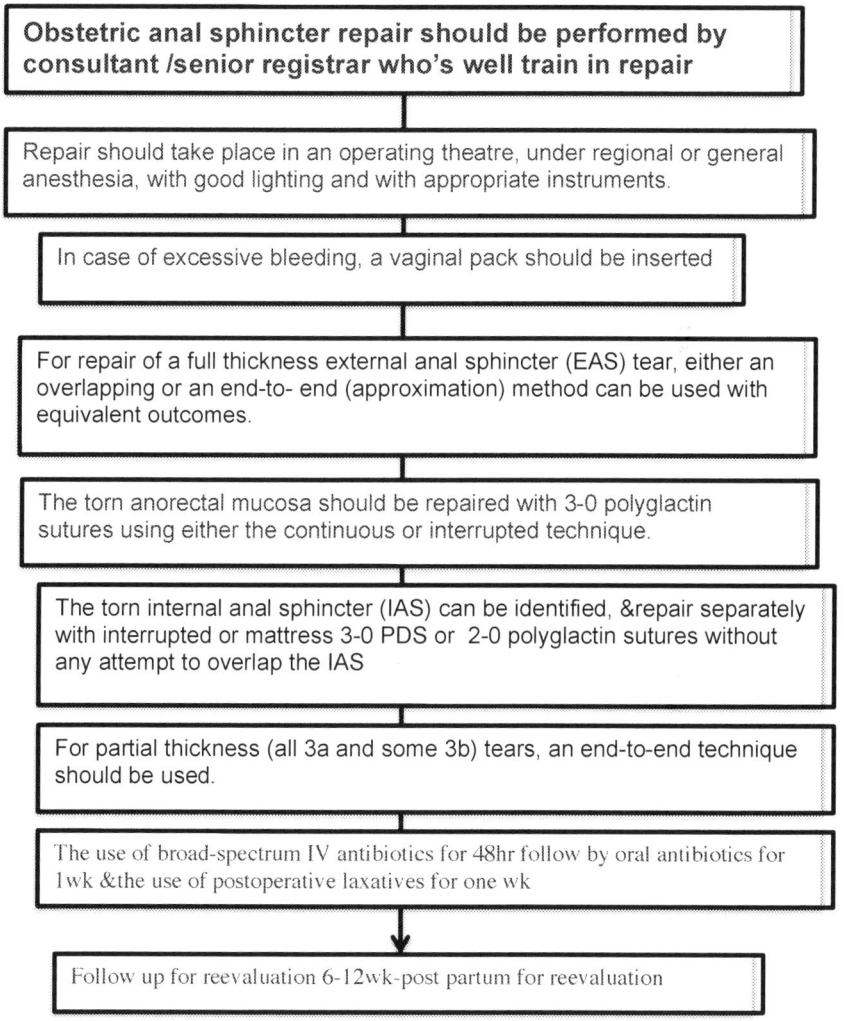

37 Labor Management of women with previous Caesarean Section in

37.1 Planned vaginal birth after ceaserian section

Vaginal birth after ceaserian section

Contraindications to VBAC

1. Women with previous uterine rupture or classical caesarean scar

2.women who have other absolute contraindications to vaginal birth that applies irrespective of the presence or absence of a scar (e.g. major placenta praevia).

3.women with complicated uterine scars, caution should be exercised and decisions should be made on a case-by-case basis by a senior obstetrician with access to the details of previous surgery.

Planned VBAC

Can be offered to a women with a singleton pregnancy with cephalic presentation at 37^{+0} weeks or beyond who have had a single previous lower segment caesarean delivery, with or without a history of previous vaginal birth.

Women who have had two or more prior lower segment caesarean deliveries may be offered VBAC after counseling by a senior obstetrician. This should include the risk of uterine rupture and maternal morbidity, and the individual likelihood of successful VBAC (e.g. given a history of prior vaginal delivery).

37.2 Labor &birth in previous Ceaserian section

Labor &birth in previous CS	1. Labour is managed to optimize a normal outcome
	2. Delivery planned at labor room with availability of obstetric theatre and onsite blood transfusion
	3. IV Access with ABO and Group & Save samples sent
	4 One to one care with midwife
	5. Continuous CTG monitoring (Fetal distress has been reported to precede uterine rupture)
	6. Meticulous monitoring of progress of labour.
	7. Concerns with progress of labour should be reported to registrar on call for labour ward.
	8. The use of Syntocinon to augment poor progress or secondary arrest must be discussed with the consultant
	9. Guideline for the use of Syntocinon in VBAC is identical to the guidelines for its use with any other labour
	10. Epidural analgesia is available on request
	11. Regular maternal observations including BP, Pulse and temperature

Awareness of classical symptoms of scar rupture - pain, scar tenderness, bleeding PV, maternal tachycardia, hypotension and fetal distress

Post partum scar palpation not required.

37.3 Induction of labor in VBAC pathway1

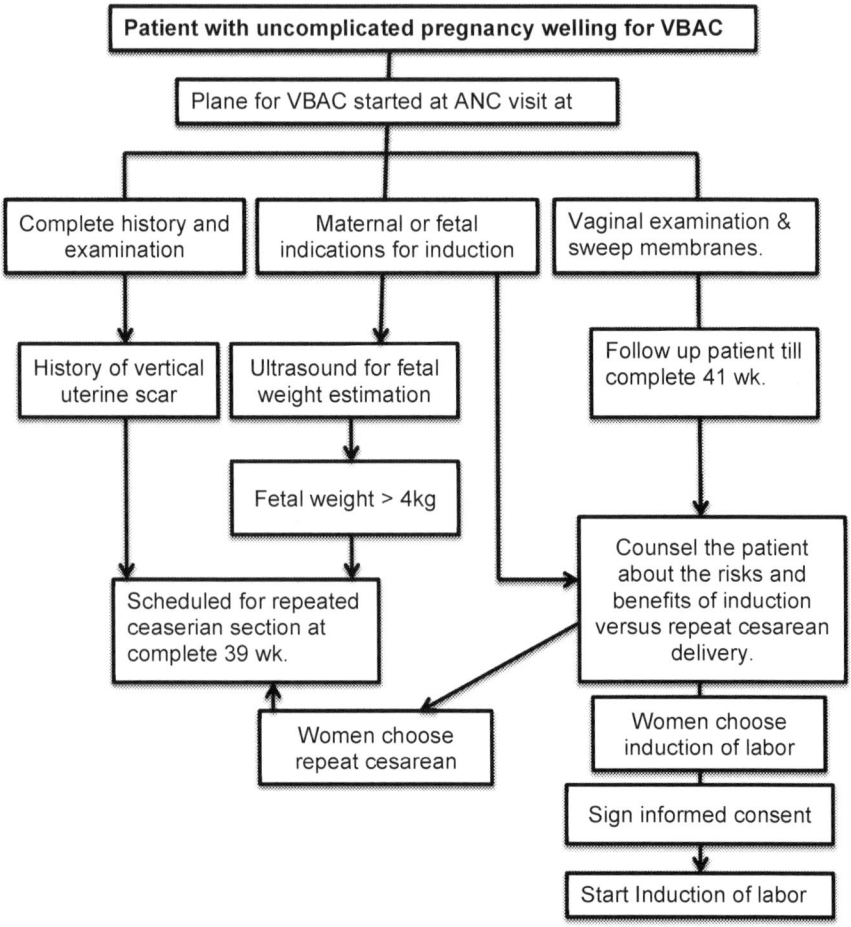

37.4 Unfavorable cervix

Induction in Unfavorable cervix previous CS

Single balloon catheter

-Under aseptic technique can use the # 16 foly catheter with balloon

Do continuous uterine activity monitoring.

Ring forceps can be used to pass a deflated balloon bladder catheter then inflate it with 60 mL NS) through the internal cervical os and into the extra amniotic space. The balloon is retracted so that it rests against the internal os.

The catheter is left in place until it is extruded or for up to 12 hours.

-Oxytocin is begun after the catheter has been extruded or removed.

A large balloon catheter may be more effective than a small one.

Intravaginal prostaglandins E2 gel

1mg every 6 hrs. for 3 doses the to be reevaluated with senior registrar/consultant on duty if not responding

Intra-vaginal prostaglandins are preferred to intra-cervical prostaglandins E2 because they results in more timely vaginal deliveries.

37.5 Favorable cervix

Induction of Favorable cervix in previous CS

Cervical ripening is unnecessary
Start with amniotomy and administration of oxytocin
A low-dose infusion oxytocin typically consists of an initial dose between 0.5 and 2.0-mill units/min, increase every 30 min till 3 regular contraction in 10 min maximumdose 32 miu

Misoprostol is not advice for induction in preveous ceaserian section

37.6 Induction of labor in previous scar pathway2

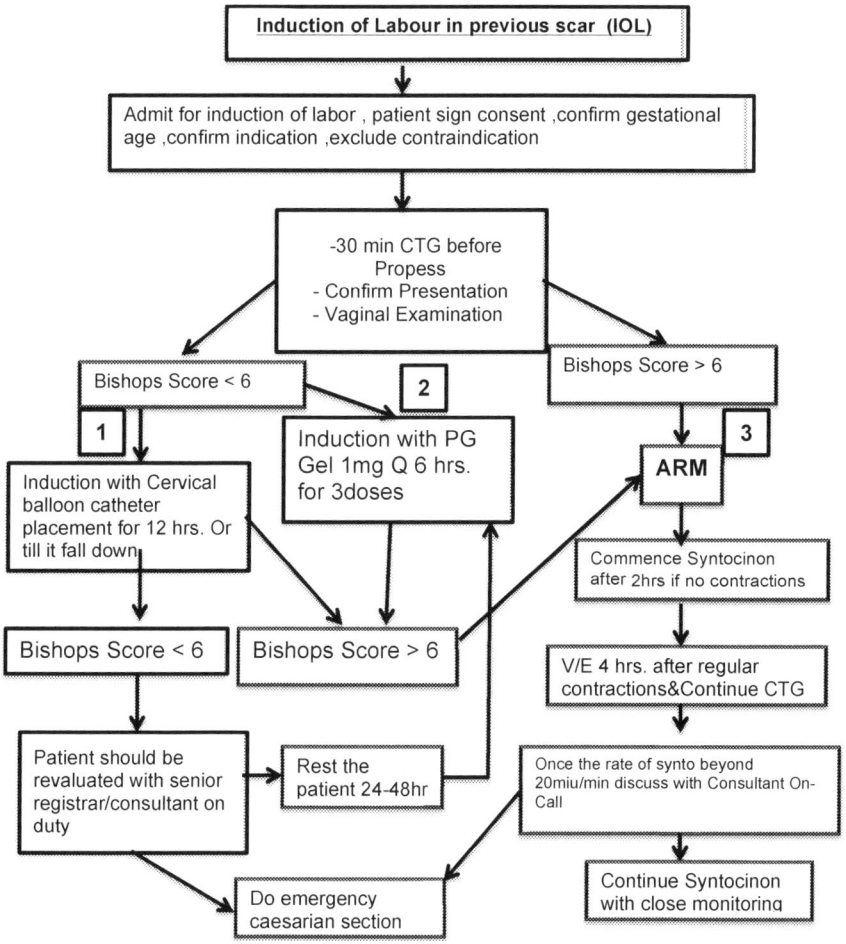

38 Spontaneous Ruptures OF Membranes (SROM)

38.1 Diagnosis

Diagnosis

1. If frank leaking no need for speculum examination
2. If it is uncertain do speculum examination
3. Avoid digital vaginal examination in the absence of contractions.

38.2 Management of SROM>37wks

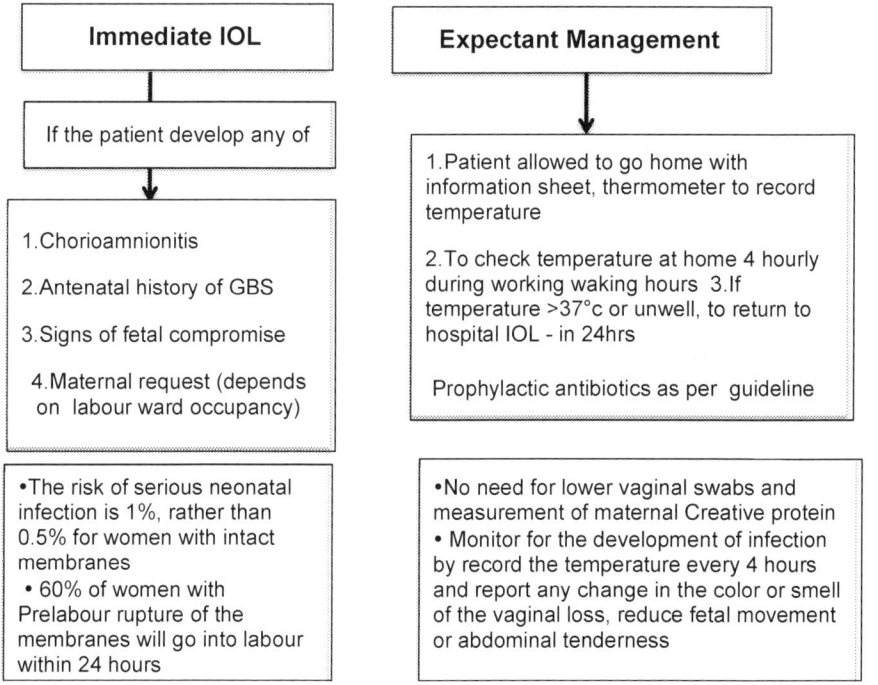

38.3 Spontaneous rupture of membrane (PPROM)<37wks pathway

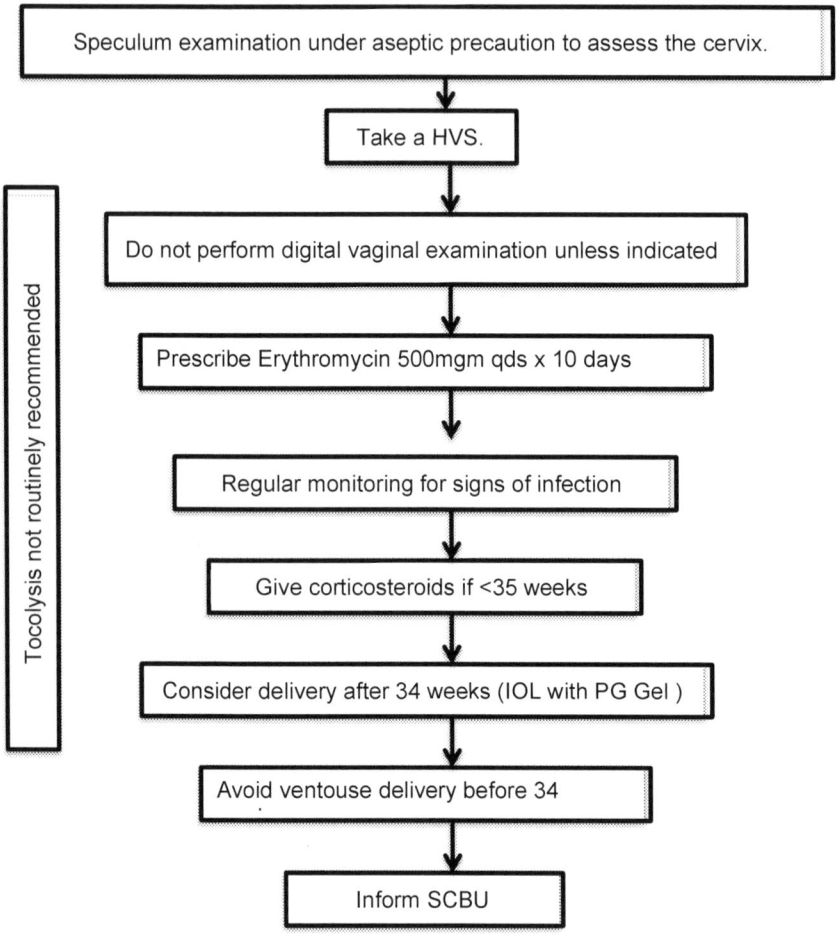

39 PRE-TERMLABOUR

39.1 Defention of preterm labour

Definition of preterm labour

Pre-term is birth of a baby less than 37 weeks of gestation age.
Associated with Painful uterine contractions occurring >1 in 10 mints with cervical effacement &dilatation.

39.2 Initial assessment

Initial assessment Threatened pre-term/pre-term labour

Pulse, temperature,
BP, urine dipstick/MSU
CTG monitoring
CBC, group & save
Abdominal exam
Scan for presentation
Speculum exam for cervical dilatation
Vaginal exam if only indicated

39.3 Pre term labor guidline

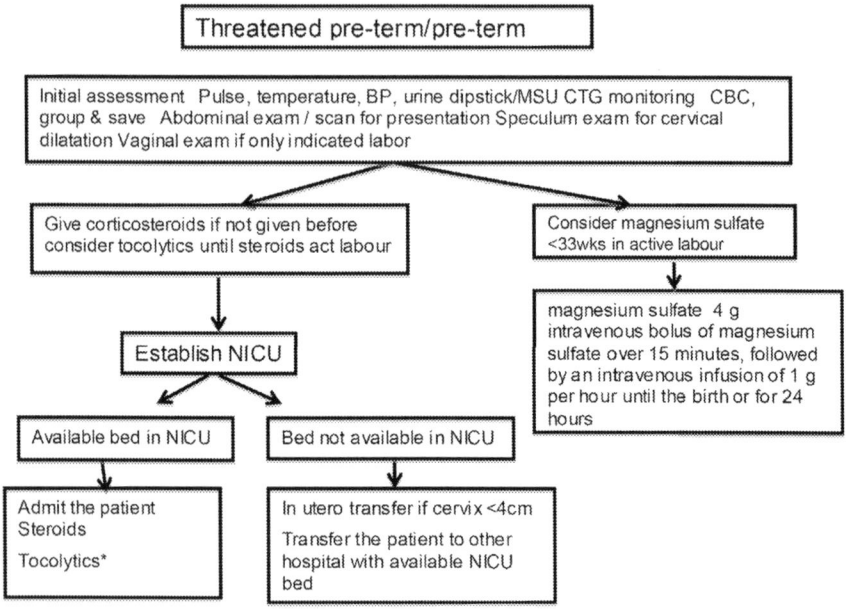

40 Corticosteroids

1.Antenatal Corticosteroids given to Reduce Neonatal Morbidity & Mortality

40.1 Indication for administration of corticosteroids

1.all women at risk of iatrogenic or spontaneous preterm birth up to 34+6 weeks of gestation.

2. all women booked for an elective caesarean section prior to 38+6 weeks of gestation.

3.donot give prophylactic steroids in women with a previous history of preterm delivery or multiple pregnancies who show no signs of being at risk of preterm birth.

4.donot give corticosteroids at gestations <24+0 weeks unless you discuss it counsultant obstetric and neonatologist

5.Antenatal corticosteroids are most effective in reducing RDS in patient deliver 24 hours after and up to 7 days after administration of the second dose of antenatal corticosteroids.

6.No reduction in neonatal death, RDS or cerebroventricular hemorrhage is seen in infants delivered more than 7 days after treatment with antenatal corticosteroids.

7.if the intial course of cortecosteriod given before 26 wks second dose can be given after the opinion of counsultant on duty

40.2 Administration of corticosteroid in special situation

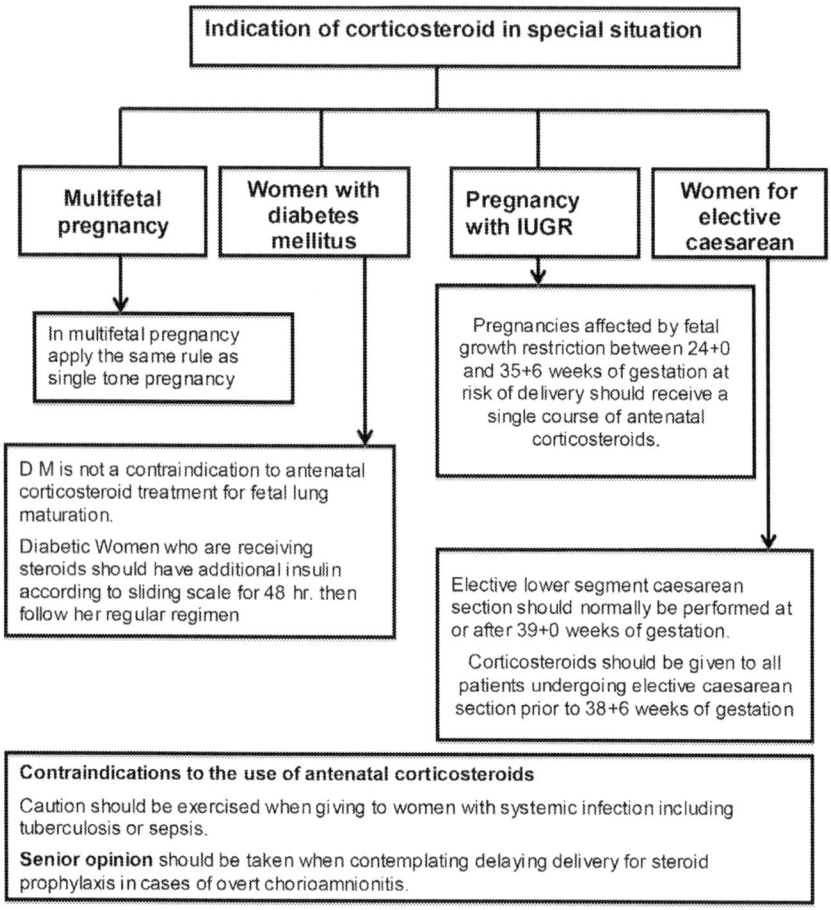

Contraindications to the use of antenatal corticosteroids

Caution should be exercised when giving to women with systemic infection including tuberculosis or sepsis.

Senior opinion should be taken when contemplating delaying delivery for steroid prophylaxis in cases of overt chorioamnionitis.

40.3 Type, dose administration corticosteroids

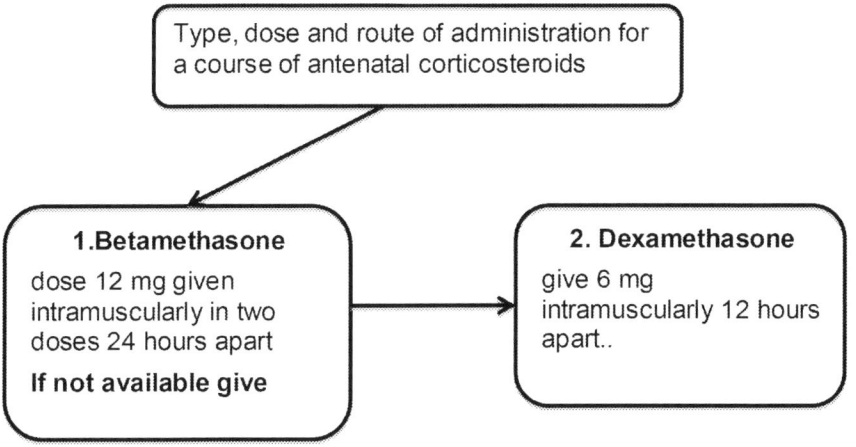

41 Tocolytics

Should be considered to complete a course of steroids or in utero transfer in case of preterm

First drug of choice

Nifedipine regime – 20mgm of oral Nifedipine as loading dose-followed

by 10- 20mgm three to four times daily, adjusted according to uterine activity up to 48hrs (total dose of 60mgm) labour
***After giving nifedipine-loading dose please check the pulse rate and BP every 30 minutes for first 2 hours then 4 hourly until next dose**

Contraindication

- Cardiogenic shock & Aortic stenosis
- Severe PET
- Intrauterine infection
- Placental abruption
- Advanced cervical dilatation
- Evidence of fetal compromise

Placental insufficiency

Relative Contraindication

- Non reassuring CTG
- IUGR
- Multiple pregnancy

Mild hemorrhage due to placenta previa

41.1 Atosiban

The choice of Atosiban (licensed) should be discussed with the duty Consultant.

Step	Regimen	Injection Rate	Atosiban dose
Bolus	Over 1 min	0.9 ml.	6.75 mg
Loading dose	3 hours	24 ml/hour	18 mg/hour (300 mcg/ min)
Maintenance dose	Up to 45 hours	8 ml/hour	6 mg/hour (100 mcg/ min)

Atosiban

Preparation

Atosiban = Tractocile = 7.5mg/ml Infusion can be given in 0.9% saline, Ringer solution, or 5% Dextrose

From a 100 ml bag, withdraw 10 ml and discard, replace it with 10 ml s Atosiban 7.5 mg/ml=75 mg in 100ml.

Loading infusion 24ml/hour=18mg/hour over 3 hours then reduce the infusion rate to 8ml/hour

- No specific antidote

Contraindications to Atosiban

>33 wks., <24 wks.,

- PROM>30 wks.
- Abnormal FH
- Placenta previa, abruption
- Severe Pre eclampsia

No data on women with abnormal liver or renal function

Theoretically increase of ph.

- No effect on lactation
- No specific antidote

42 Hypertensive disease in pregnancy

42.1 Definitions of HTN disease in pregnancy

Hypertensive disease in pregnancy

Mild Hypertension

BP 140-149/90-99 mmHg

Severe hypertension

BP ≥ 160/110 mmHg with multisystem involvement

Aim of the therapy is to keep BP < 150/80-100 mmHg

42.2 Preeclampsia definition

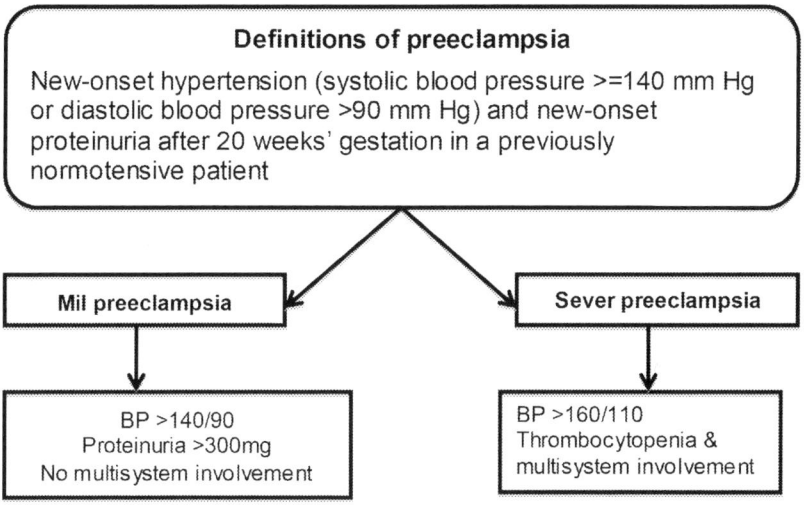

Hypertension	Proteinuria	Multisystem Involvement
>140 mm Hg systolic or >90 mm Hg diastolic	>300 mg in 24 h	Thrombocytopenia
Previously normotensive patient >20 wk. gestation	Protein/creatinine ratio >=0.3 mg/dl	Renal insufficiency
BP measured two times at least 4 hours apart	Dipstick 11 (only if other methods not available)	Liver dysfunction
		Pulmonary edema
		Cerebral or visual disturbances

42.3 Preeclampsia management pathway

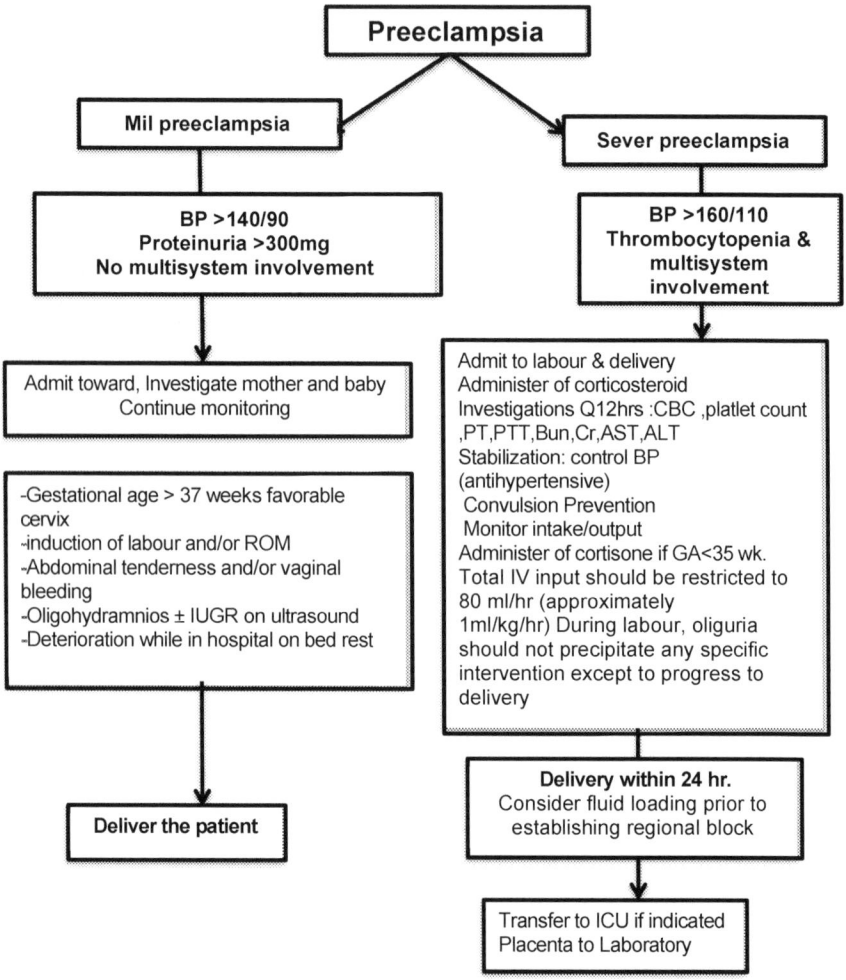

42.4 Features of Severe preeclampsia

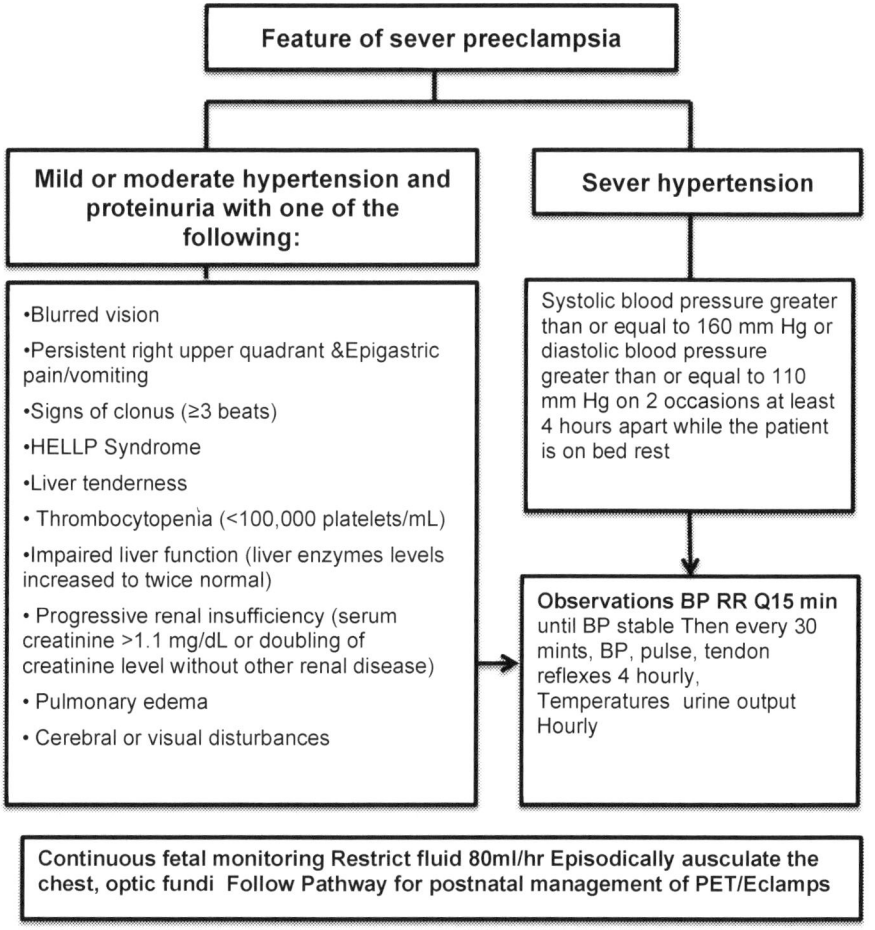

43 Eclampsia

43.1 Eclampsia management pathway

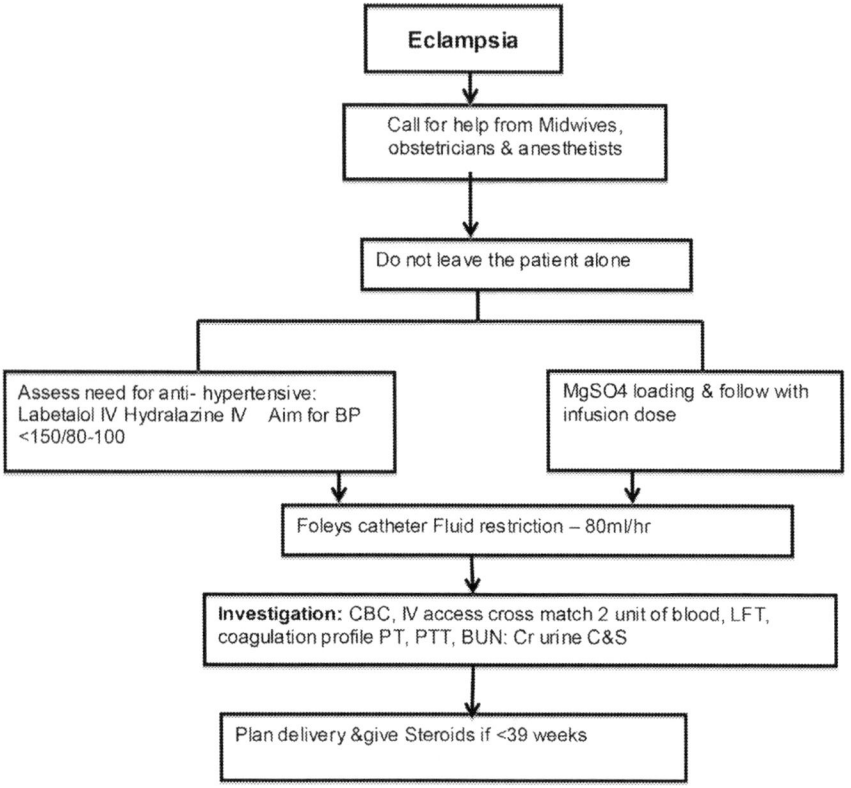

43.2 Recurrence of seizures management pathway

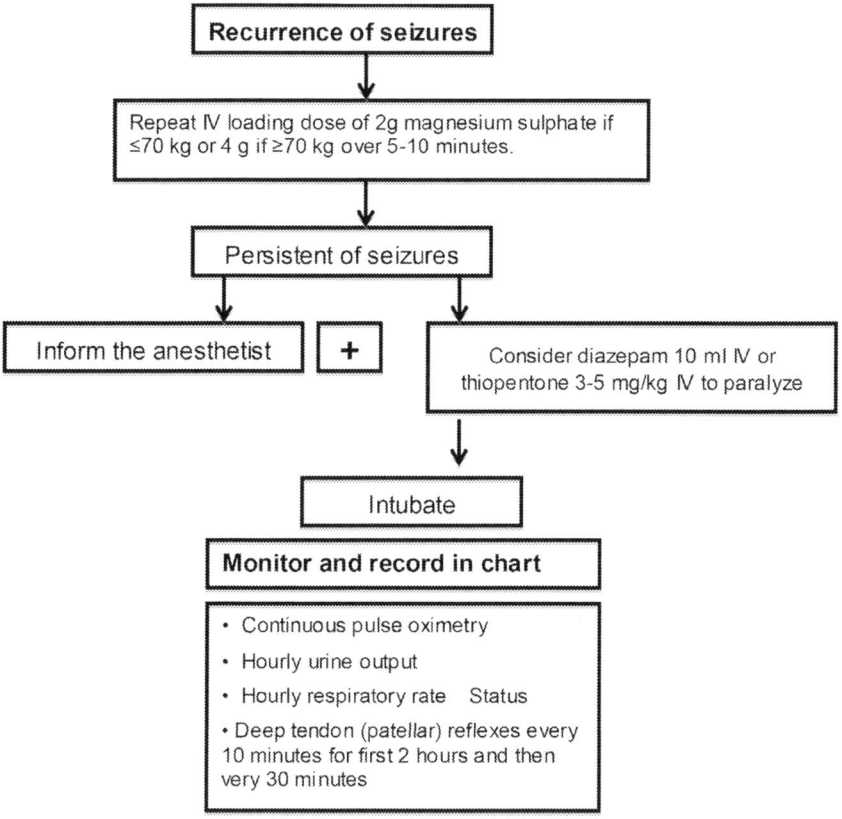

Stop magnesium sulphate infusion and check the levels

If

Urine output is < 100 ml in 4 hours

- Patellar reflexes are absent (assuming not due to regional block)
- Respiratory rate < 16 beats/ minute
- O_2 saturation is < 90% There is no need to measure magnesium levels if urine output is maintained Check magnesium levels if toxicity is suspected on clinical grounds

The antidote of magnesium toxicity is 10ml of 10% calcium gluconate –slow IV Restart the magnesium sulphate if urine output improve

Management of sever preeclampsia

Admit to labor word

Inform senior pediatrician &anesthesiologist on call

Inform senior obstetrician on call

Request PET investigation

Start Magnesium sulphate protocol

Start antihypertensive agent

Continuous close monitoring 24-48 hrs

43.3 Post Partum Fluid Protocol – Pre Eclampsia

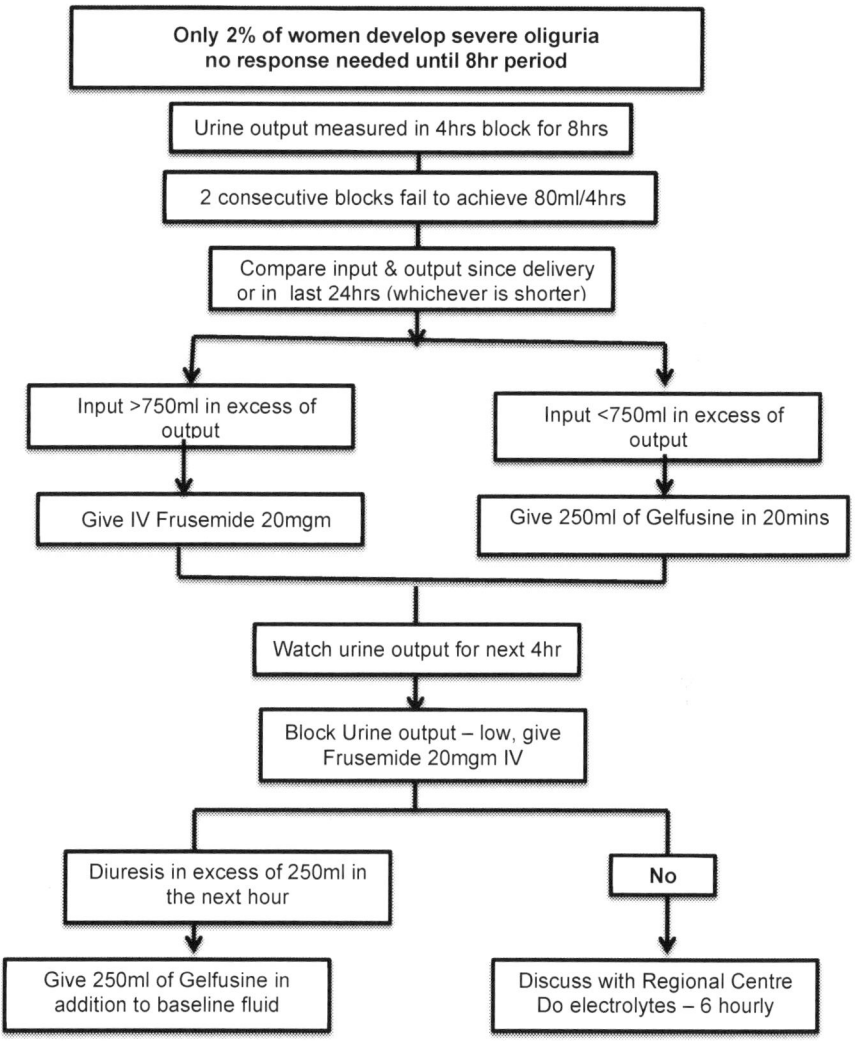

43.4 Anti hypertensive

Aim of the therapy is to keep BP<150/80-100mmHg

43.5 Choice of antihypertensive

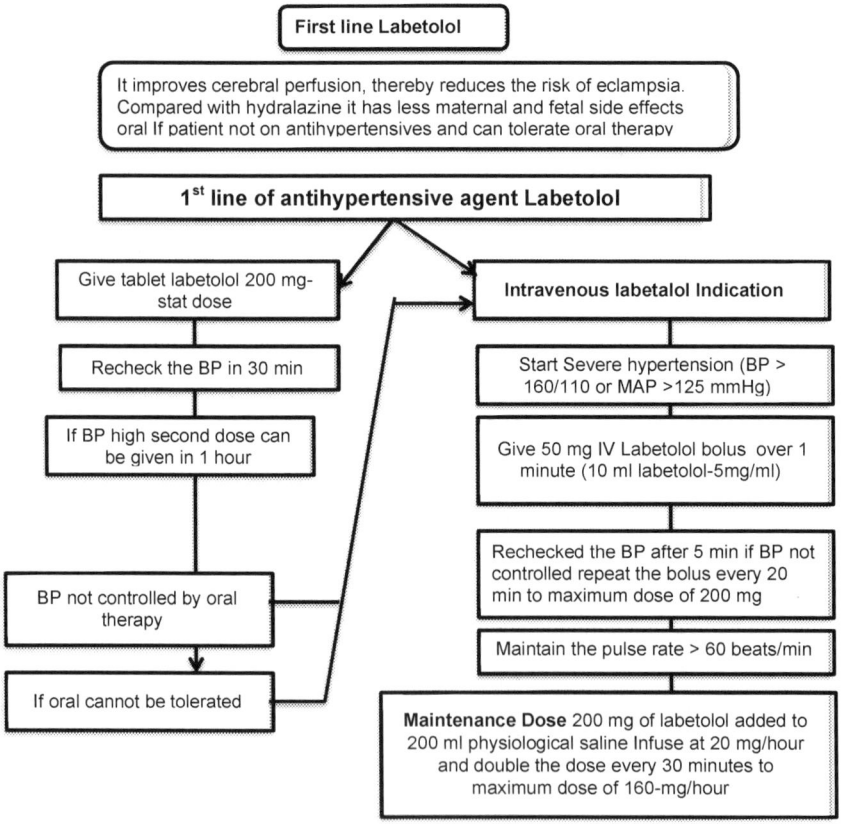

43.6 2nd line of antihypertensive agent pathway

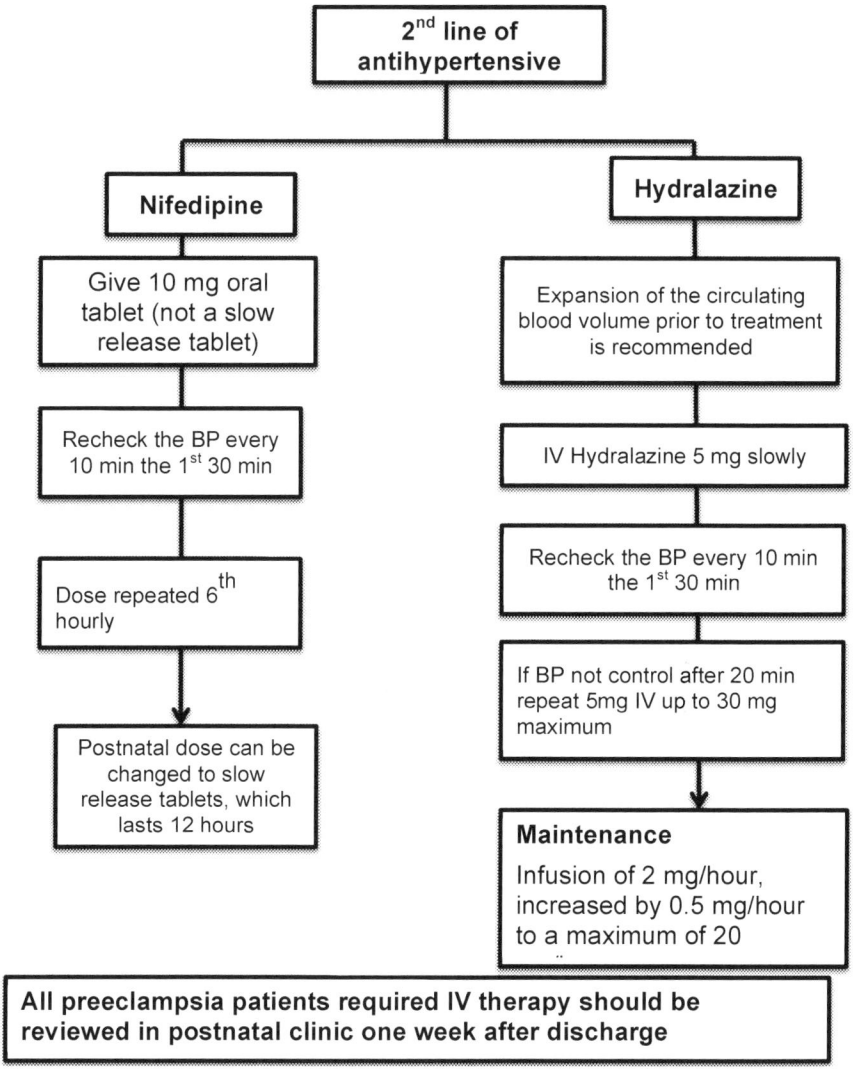

43.7 Seizure prophylaxis Magnesium sulphate protocol

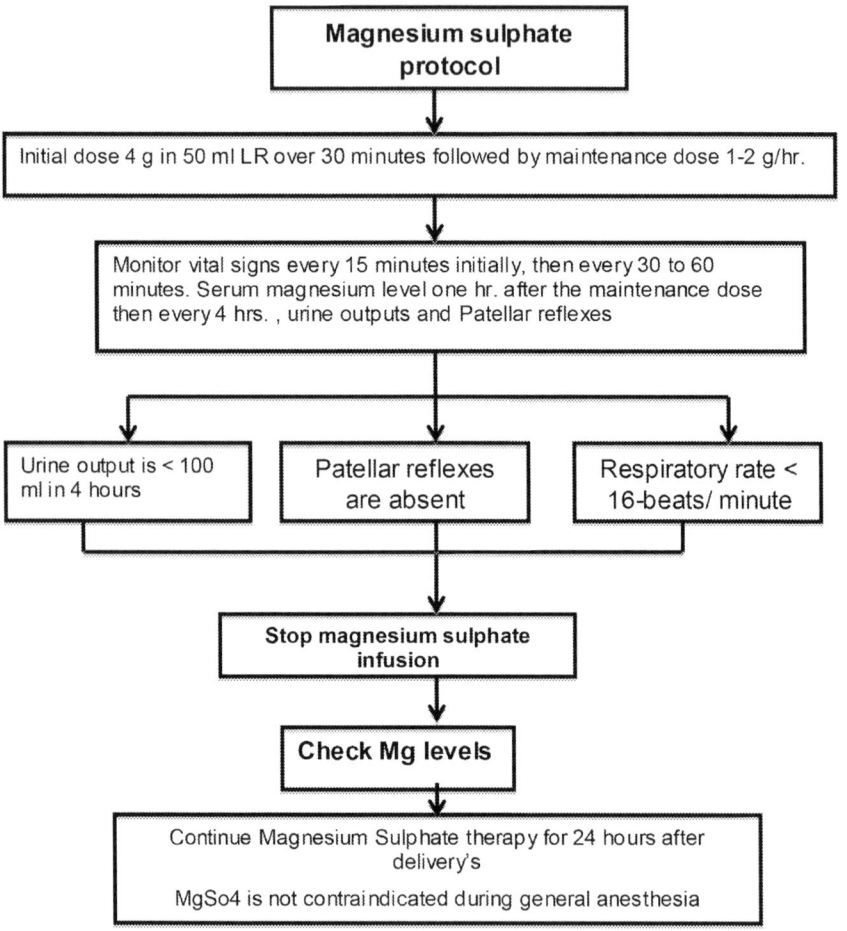

43.8 Treatment Of Magnesium Toxicity

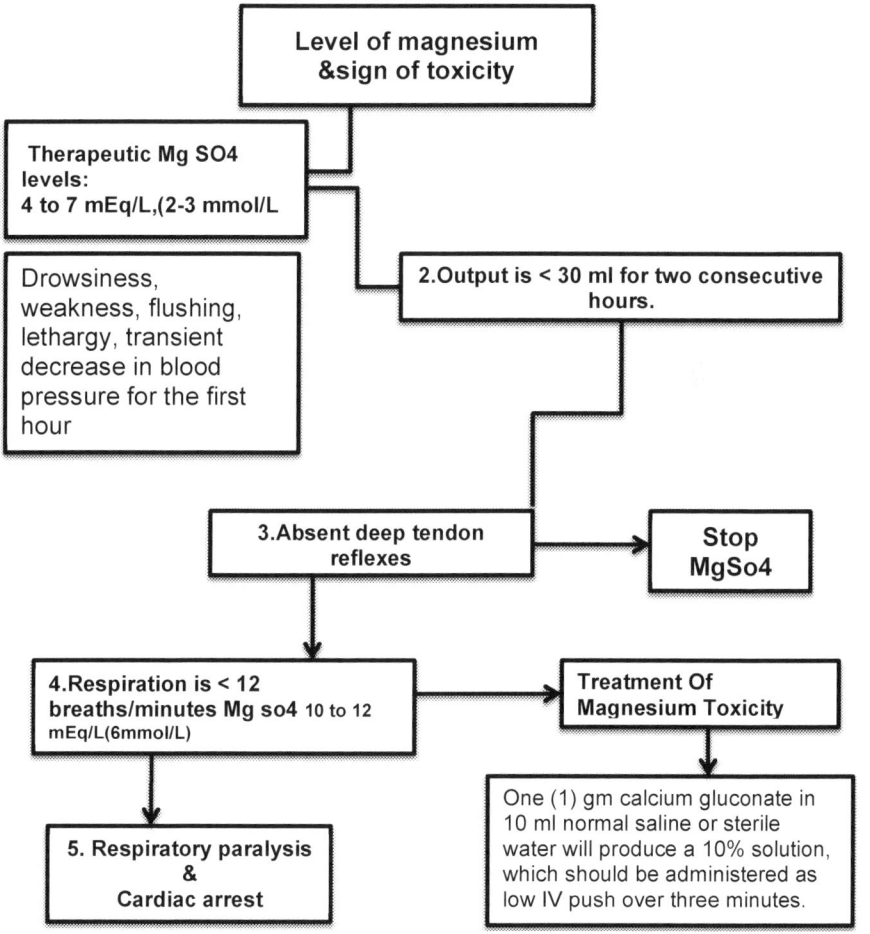

44 Management of Laboring Women with IDDM/Gestational Diabetes

44.1 Time of delivery

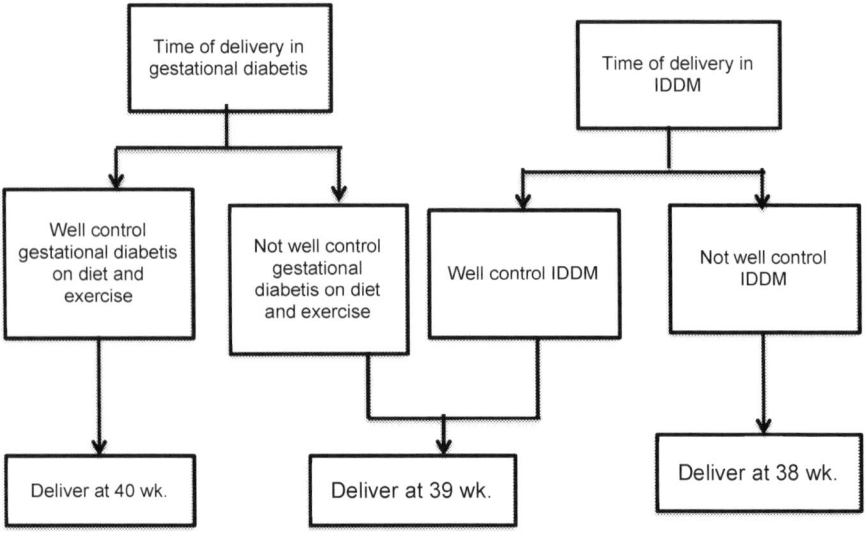

44.2 Methods of delivery

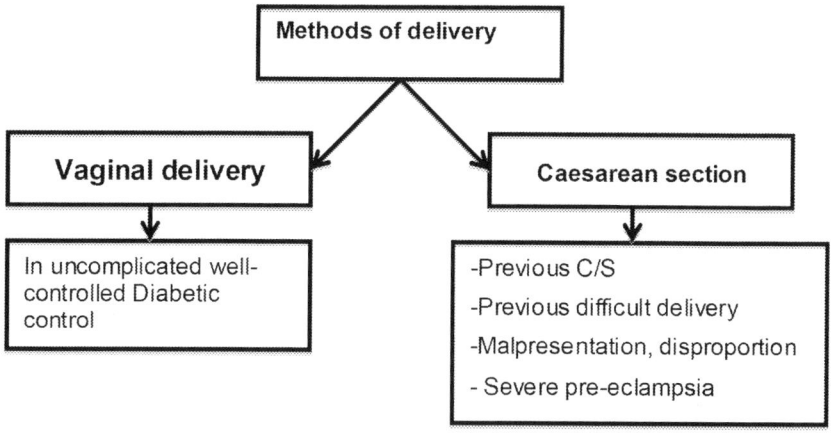

44.3 Control of blood glucose during latent phase of labor

Control of blood glucose during latent phase

1.patient is on her usual diet

2.follow SQ insulin protocol

3.Blood glucose monitoring: fasting, 2 hours post prandial

If uncontrolled call the endocrine team (above target or hypoglycemic attack)

44.4 Control of blood glucose during during active phase &NPO for elective ceaserian section

Control of blood glucose during during active phase &NPO for elective ceaserian section

1. Start IV insulin infusion+ IV fluid and KCL infusion as in protocol (order by endocrine/internal medicine team)
2.follow serum electrolytes as per protocol.
3.transfer patient to labour ward.
4.follow blood glucose hourly call endocrine /internal medicine team if blood glucose >10mmmol/L or <4 mmol/L
5.inform obstetric &anesthesia registrar.
6.start high-risk monitoring –maternal observations, continuous CTG, maintenance of partogram
7.keep senior obstetrician on call informed about progress. Anticipate shoulder dystocia at birth and follow protocol for shoulder dystocia

44.5 Diabetic patient Post delivery pathway

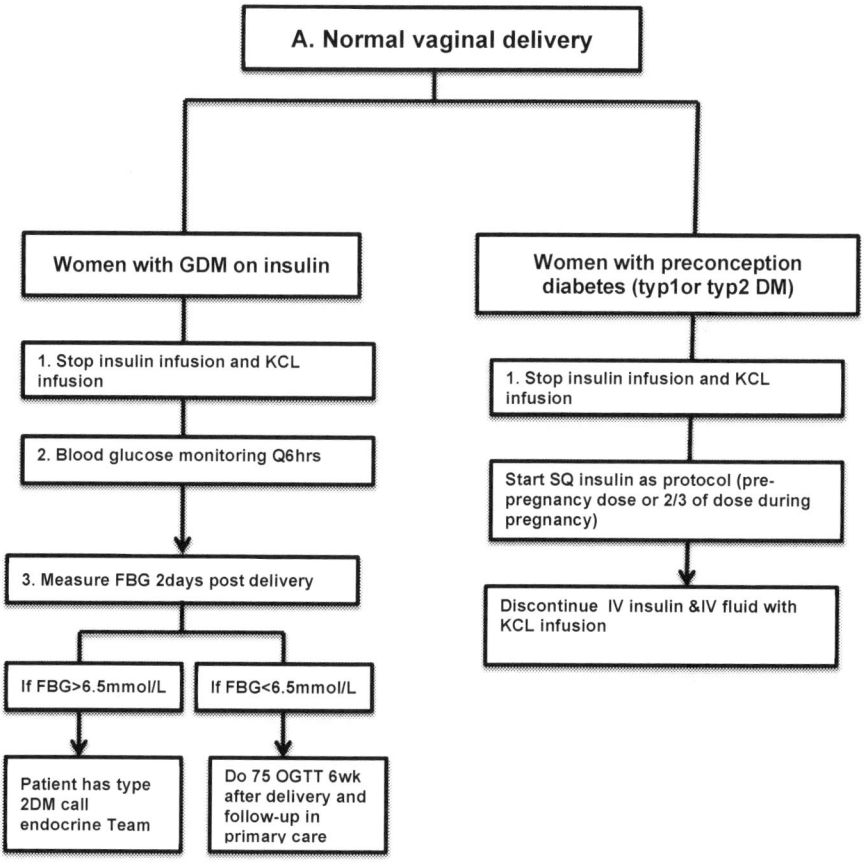

44.6 Diabetic patient on insulin with preterm labor

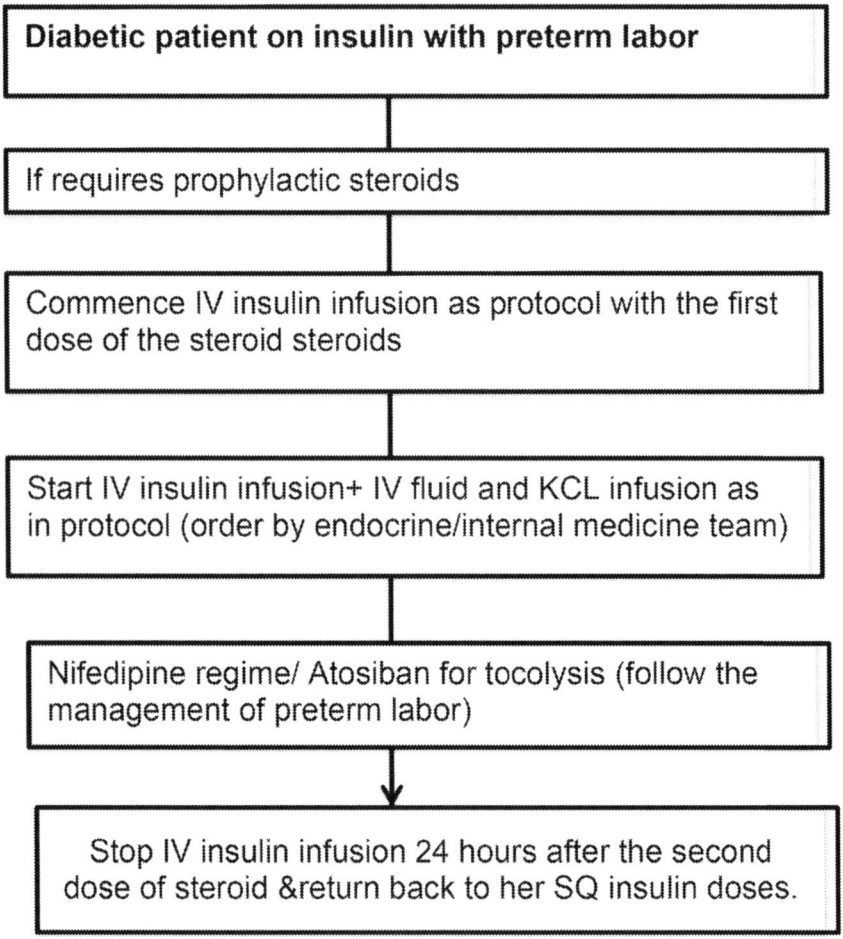

44.7 Diabetic pregnant women with KDA

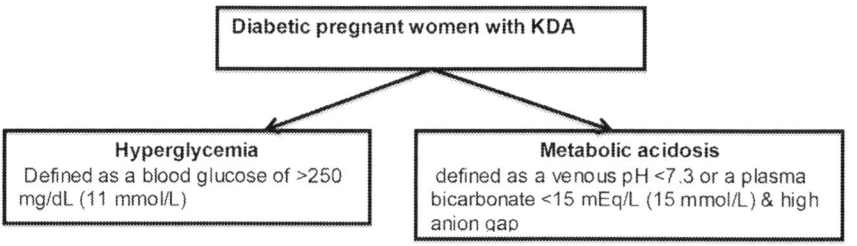

44.8 Management of DKA

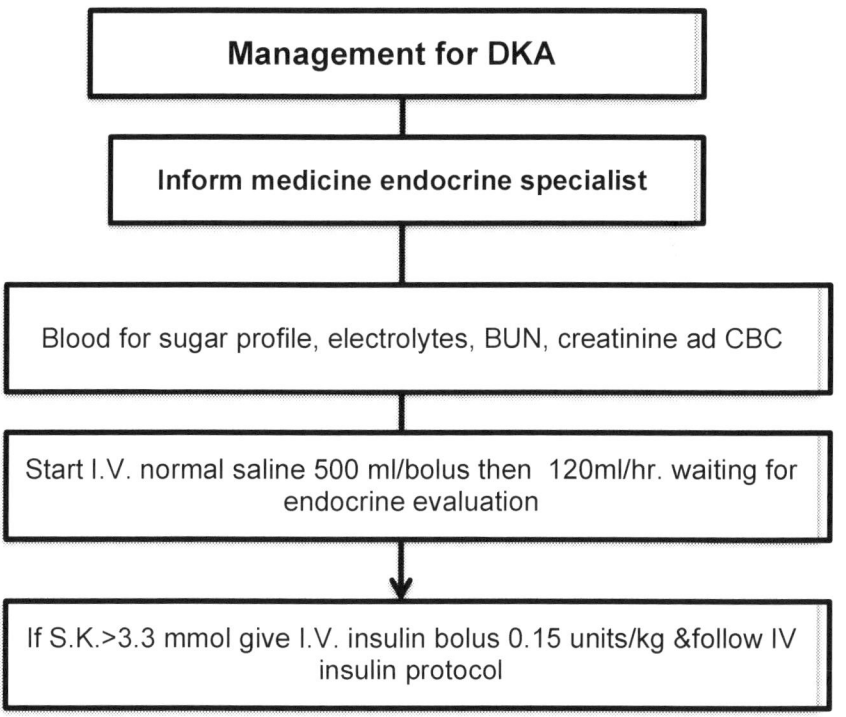

45 Antepartum Hemorrhage

45.1 Classification of the severity of APH.

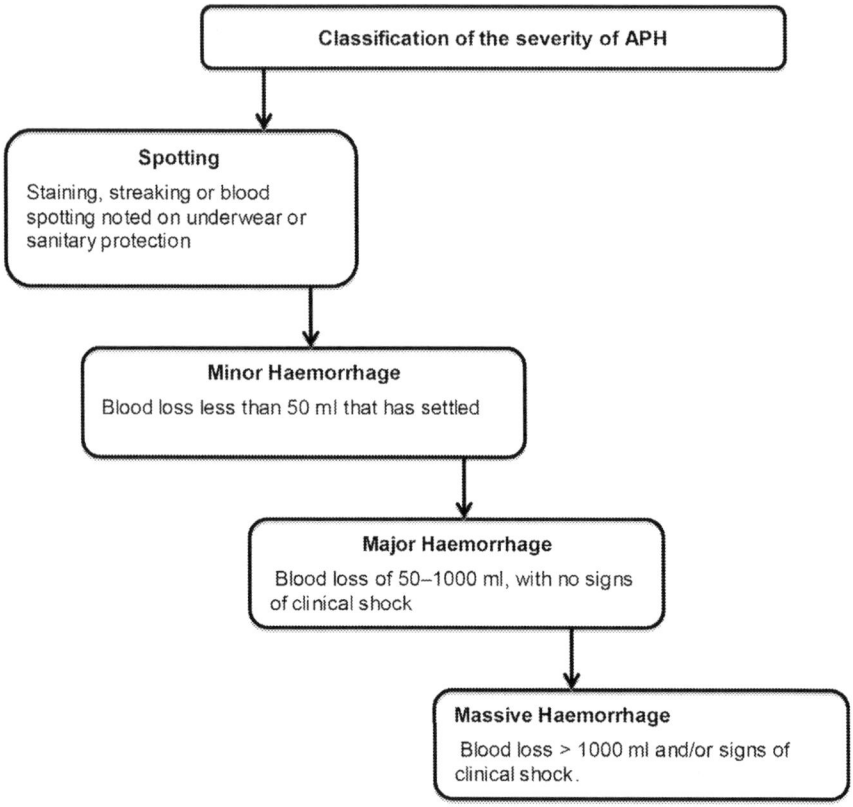

45.2 Causes Antepartum haemorrhage

Causes Antepartum haemorrhage

1.placental abruption
2.placenta praevia
3.vasa praevia
4.obstetric haemorrhage
5.obstetric hemorrhage

45.3 Complications of APH

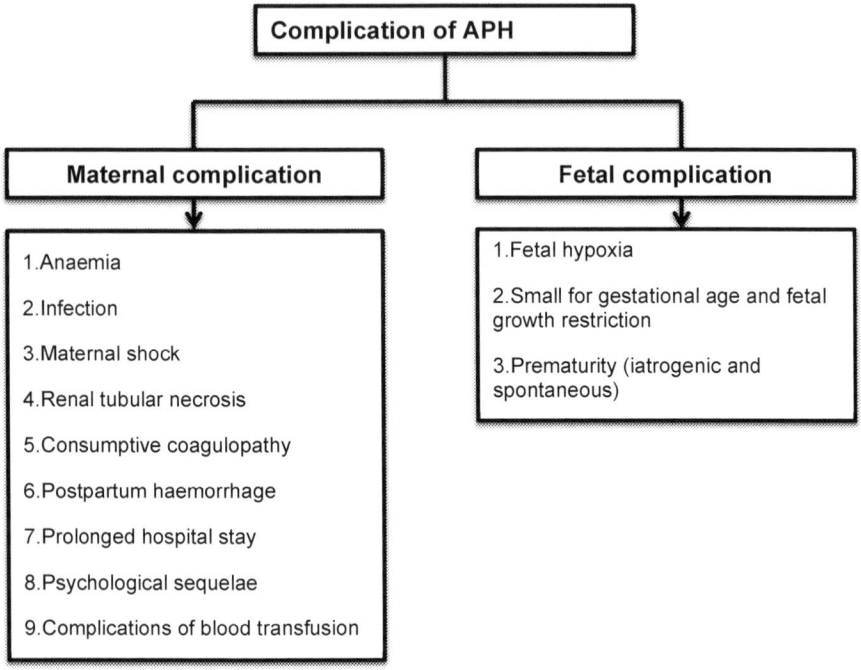

45.4 The main therapeutic goal of management of massive blood loss:

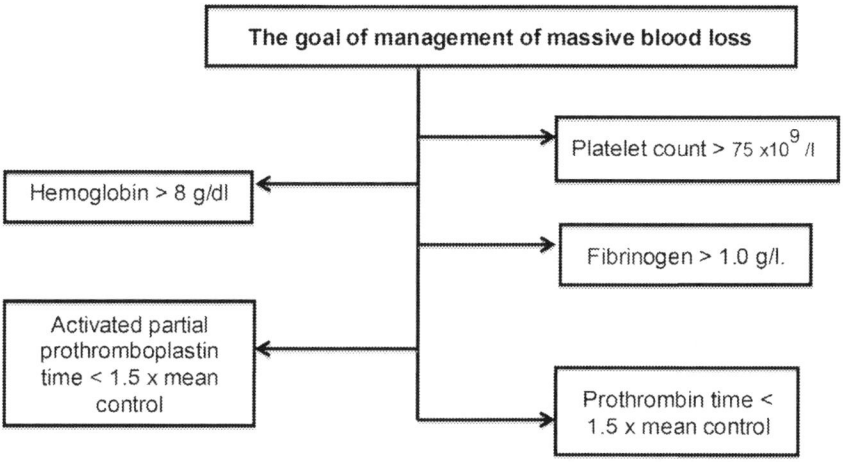

45.5 Fluid therapy and blood product transfusion

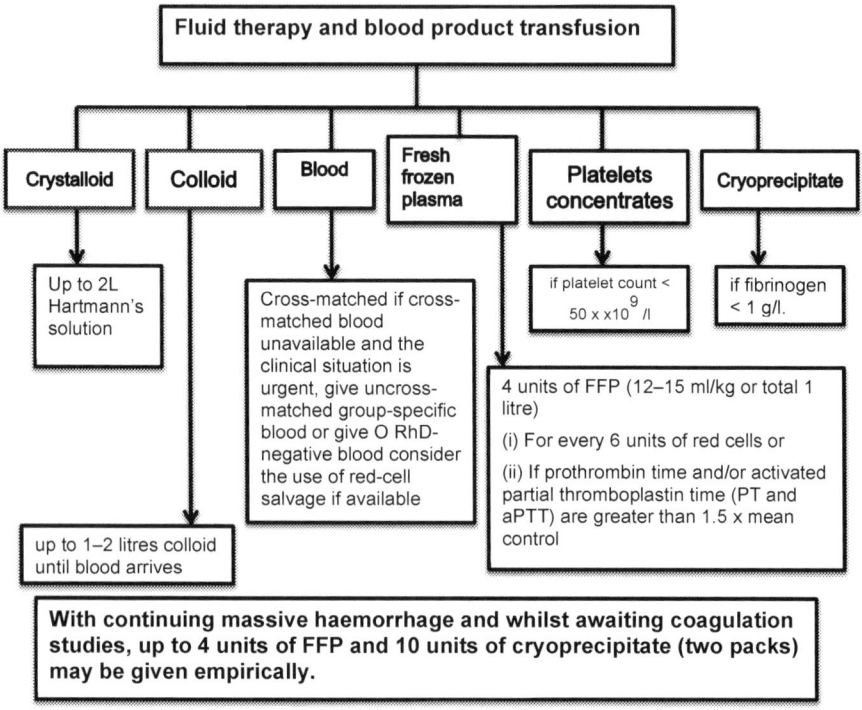

45.6 Antepartum Hemorrhage pathway

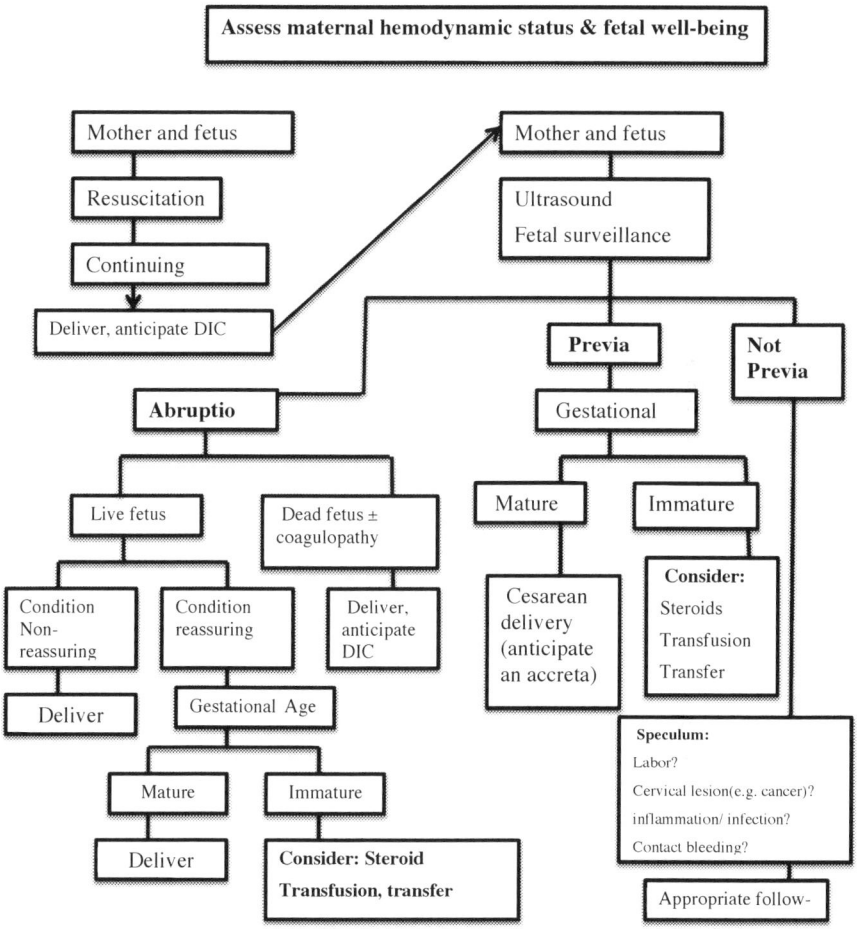

46 Genital Herpes during pregnancy

46.1 Protocol for Genital Herpes during Labour or <34 weeks gestation

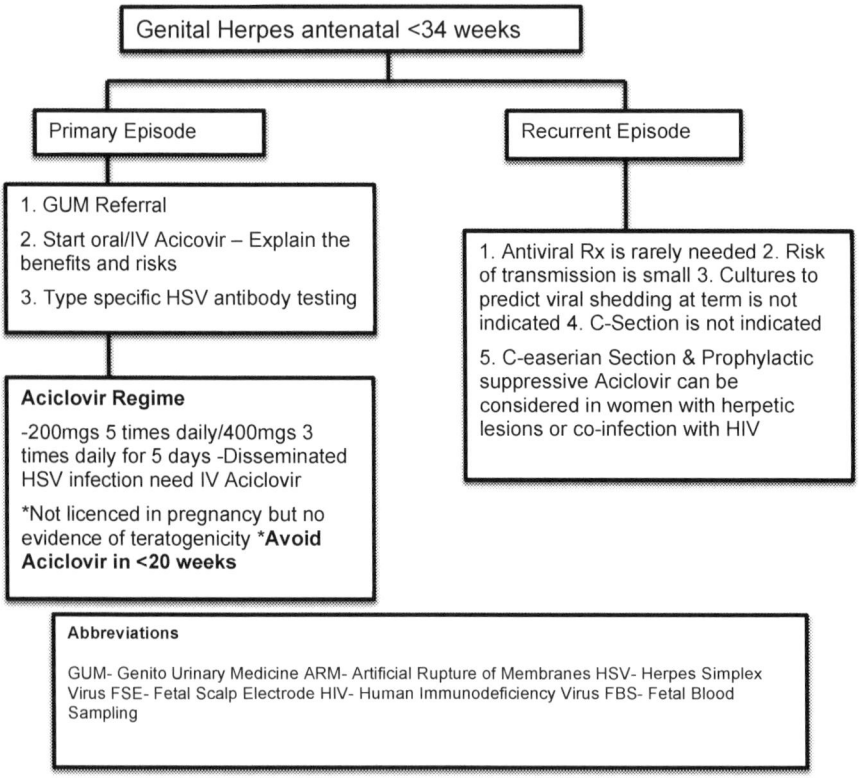

46.2 Protocol for Genital Herpes during Labour or >34 weeks gestation

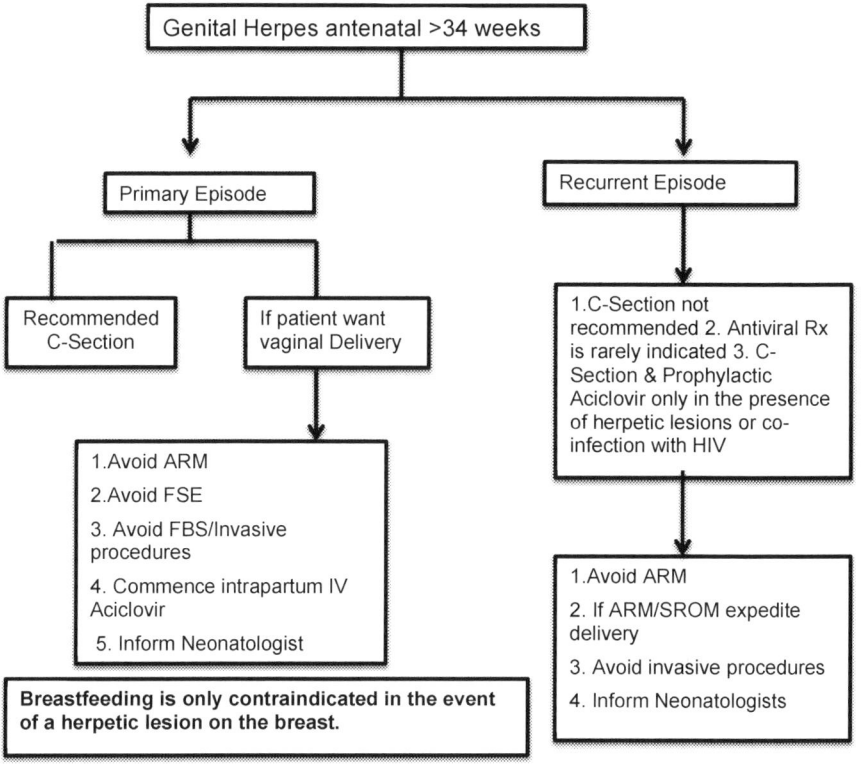

47 Instrumental delivery pre-requisites

47.1 Pre-requisites for instrumental vaginal delivery

Pre-requisites for instrumental vaginal delivery

Cervix is fully dilated

Fetal head should not be palpable abdominally

Vertex should be at or below spines (0 station) – not caput

Ensure exact position of fetal head

Check mother understands and agrees with the plan.

Written consent taken for trial in theatre

Ensure analgesia Pudendal block/Epidural/Spinal

Inform Neonatologists to attend delivery

Consultant /Senior (registrar/resident) will decide if instrumental delivery is to be conducted and senior obstetrician should present at the time of conducting instrumental delivery

47.2 Instrumental delivery application pathway

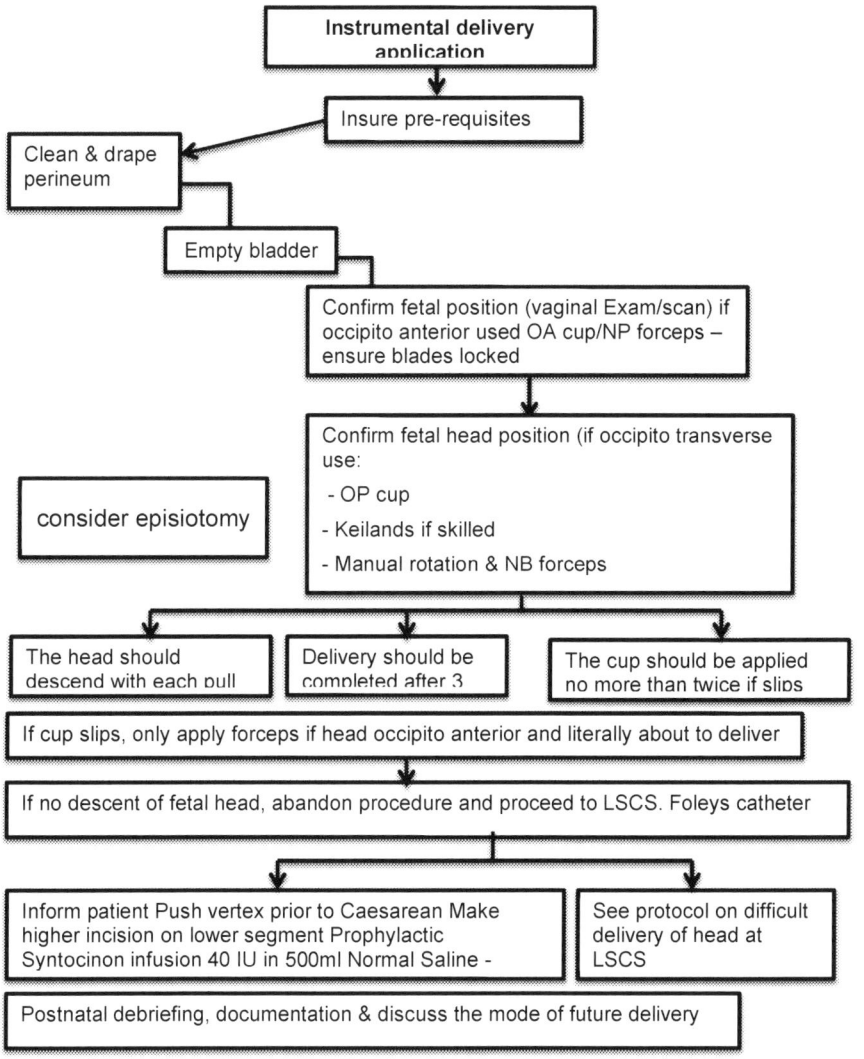

48 Pre Requisites for Caesarean Section guideline

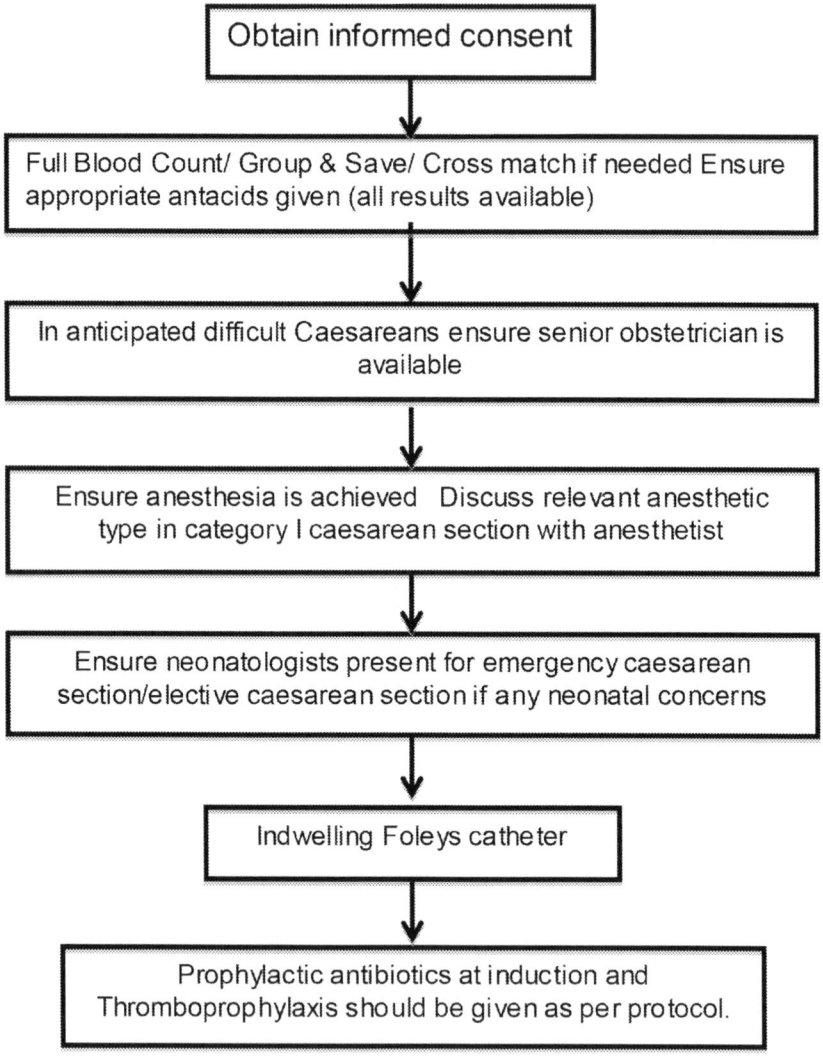

49 Caesarean Section

49.1 Classification Of Caesarean Sections

Category	Time	Definition
1A	30 min	Immediate threat to life of women or fetus, e.g. cord prolapse, uterine rupture, pathological CTG mandate immediate action
IB	30-60 min	Maternal/fetal compromise which is not immediately life-threatening, e.g. APH, failure to progress with maternal or fetal compromise
2	1-6hr	No maternal or fetal compromise but needs early delivery (scheduled) e.g. failed IOL or failure to progress
3		Delivery timed to suit the woman or staff (elective)

49.2 second Stage Caesarean Section pathway

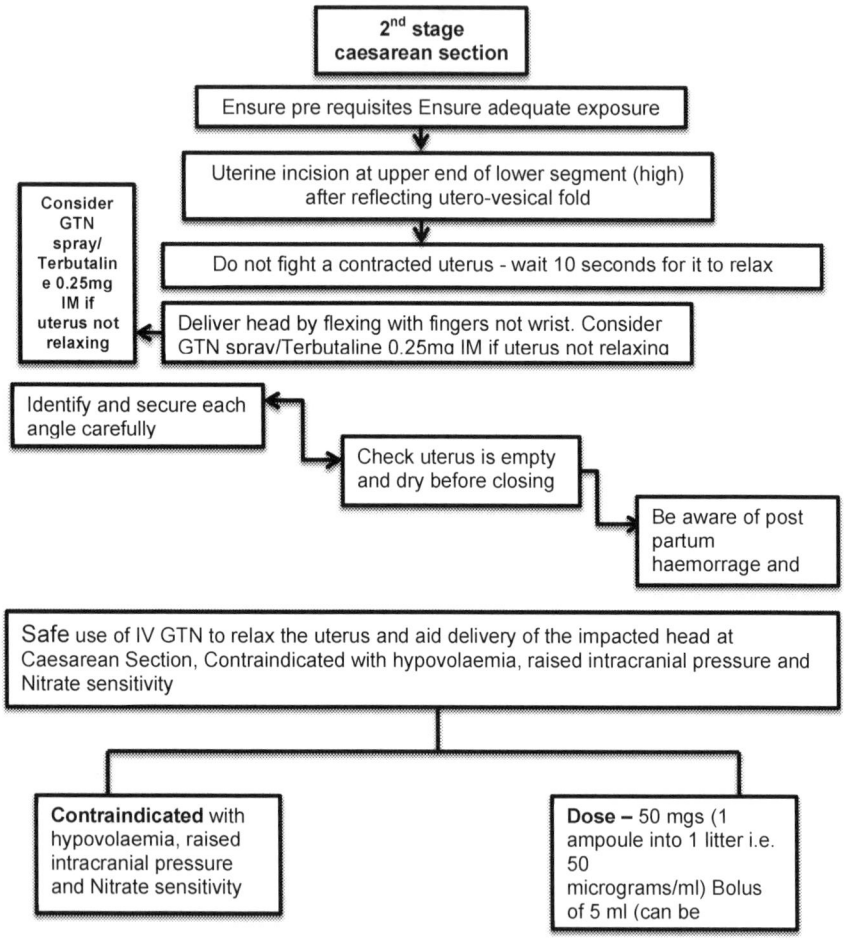

49.3 Prophylactic Antibiotics

Prophylactic Antibiotics

Cefuroxime 1.5g IV on call for Operation Theater

Cefazolin (1 g if ≤60 kg, 2 g for >60 kg) on call for Operation Theater

Ampicillin (2 g)IV on call for operation theater

If patient allergic to pencillin

Metronidazole (500 mg) + gentamicin (1.5 mg/kg) single dose with umbilical cord clamp Or

Clindamycin (600 mg) plus gentamicin (1.5 mg/kg) single dose with umbilical cord clamp

50 Breech Delivery

Breech in labour

-Council the patient regarding the mode of delivery by the senior registrar
-Confirm the presentation by ultrasound
-Delivery should be conducted by expert regestrsr, senior registrar
- An Anaesthetist and Paediatrician should be present at the delivery.
-Discuss the use of syntocinon if needed with consultant

50.1 Management of Breech Presentation in laboring pathway (Expected and Unexpected Breech)

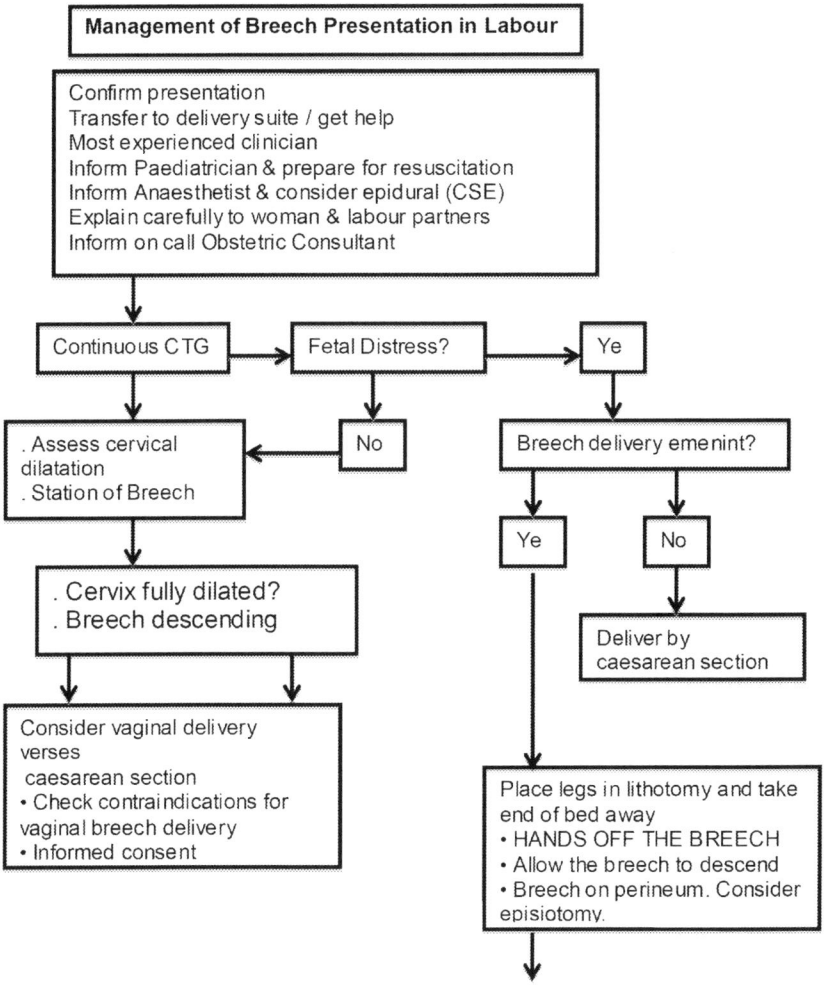

Place legs in lithotomy and take end of bed away
- HANDS OFF THE BREECH
- Allow the breech to descend
- Breech on perineum. Consider episiotomy.

↓

Place legs in lithotomy and take end of bed away
- HANDS OFF THE BREECH
- Allow the breech to descend
- Breech on perineum. Consider episiotomy.

↓

With further descent, legs usually deliver without handling.
- If delay with extended legs, deliver by flexion at knee joint and extension at hips
- DO NOT ALLOW BABY'S BACK TO ROTATE POSTERIORLY
- BABY'S SACRUM MUST BE UPPERMOST IF WOMAN IS SUPINE
- Allow arms to deliver.
- If arms extended and delaying progress, LOVSETT'S manoeuvre
- Allow breech and head to descend until the nape of the neck is visible

↓

Mauriceau-Smellie Veit manoeuvre Breech Trouble Shooting.
- Forceps, if required, by skilled obstetrician

50.2 Complecated breech delivery pathway

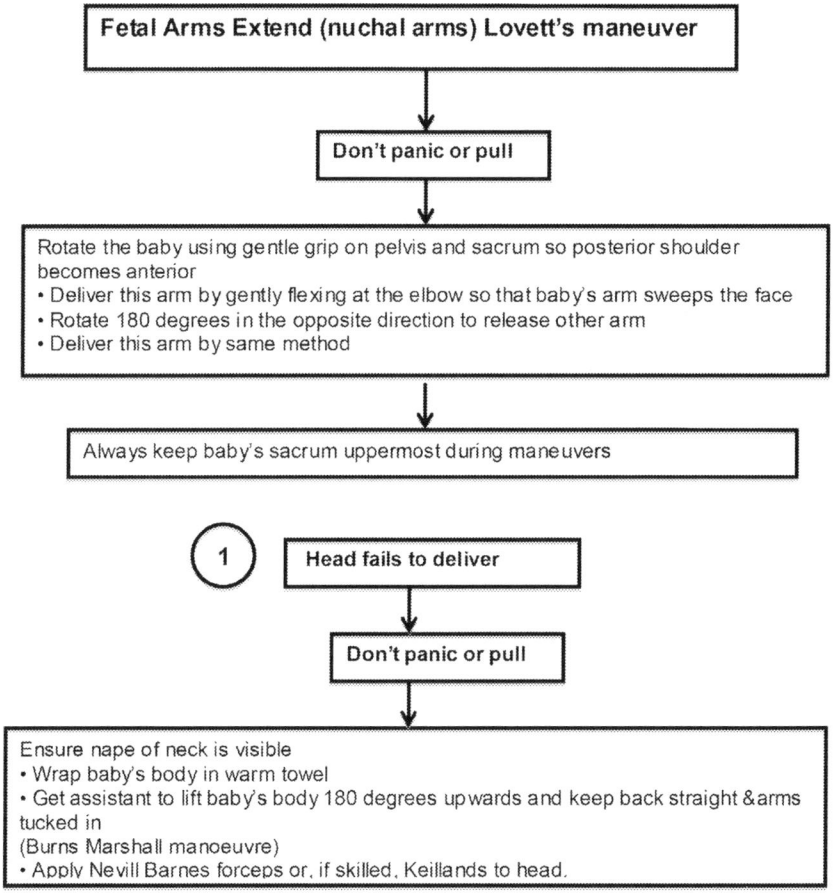

51 Twin Delivery

51.1 Twin management pathway

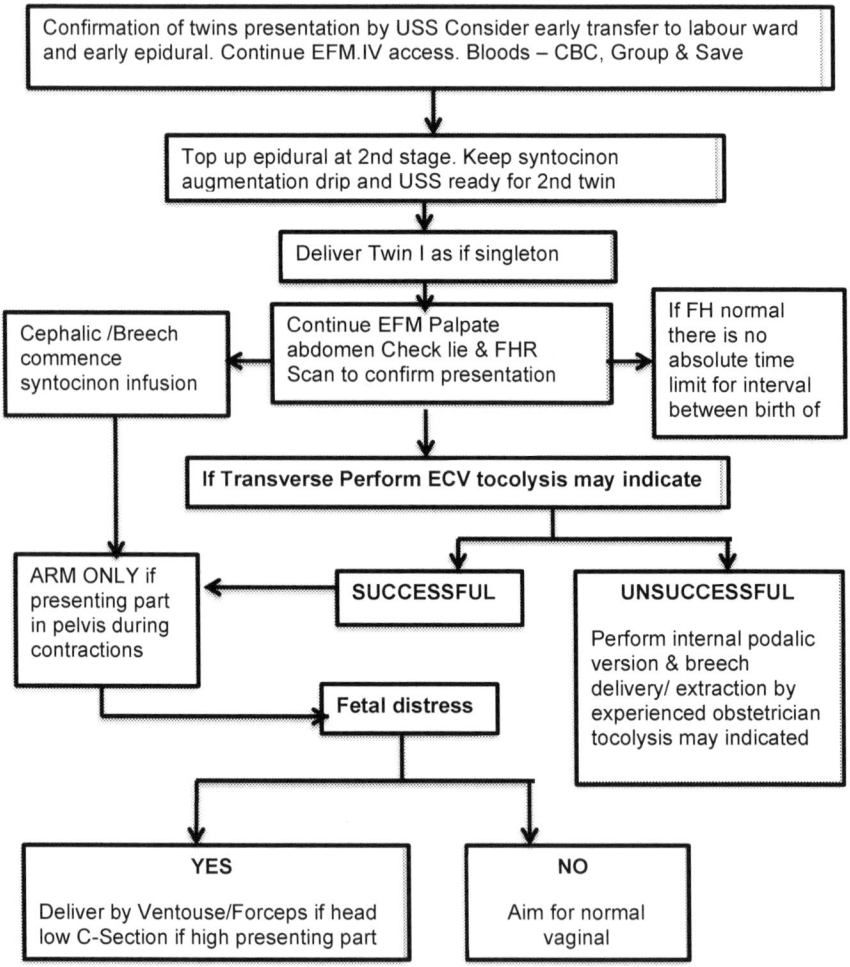

51.2 Twin delivery Management pathway

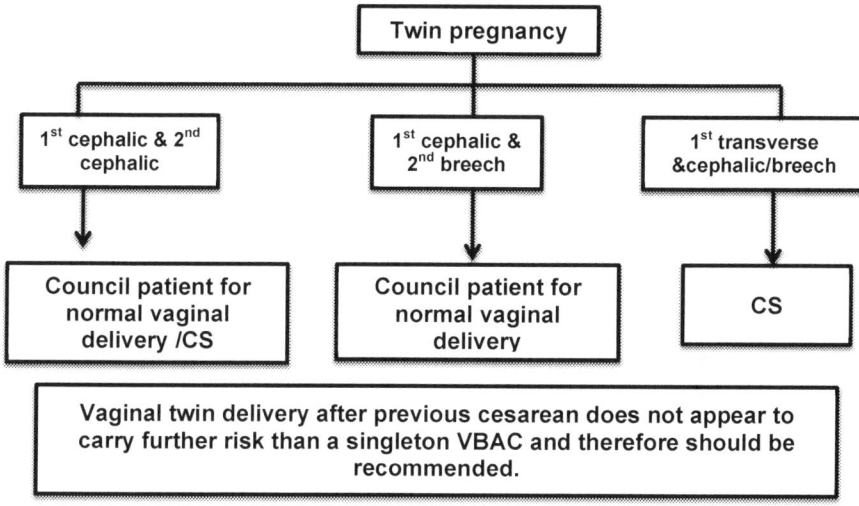

51.3 Analgesia

Analgesia

1.1 Maternal choice is of key importance and all options be considered. Epidural is the method of choice.

-The benefit of effective epidural it allows rapid top-up for a trial of instrumental delivery, external or internal version of the second twin or CS if there are problems.

-The anesthetist should be aware of the progress of labour
-Elective epidural top-up for the delivery of the second twin will facilitate manipulation, instrumental delivery and rapid top-up for CS.

52 Shoulder Dystocia management pathway

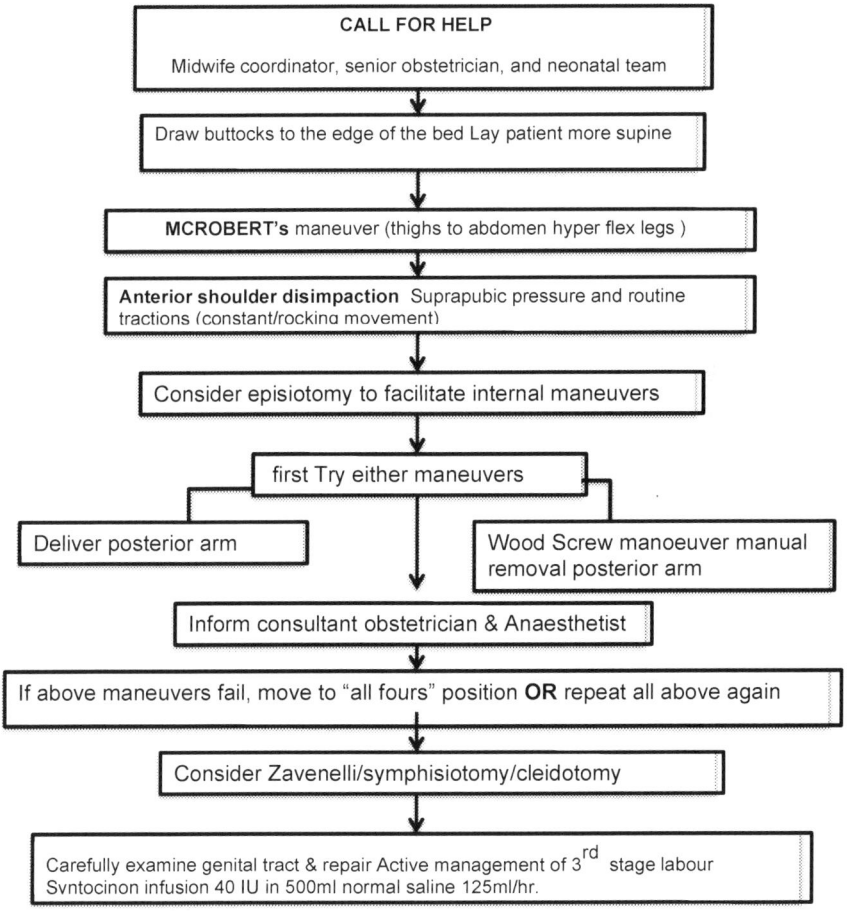

53 Management of Cord Prolapse

53.1 Definitions Cord Presentation

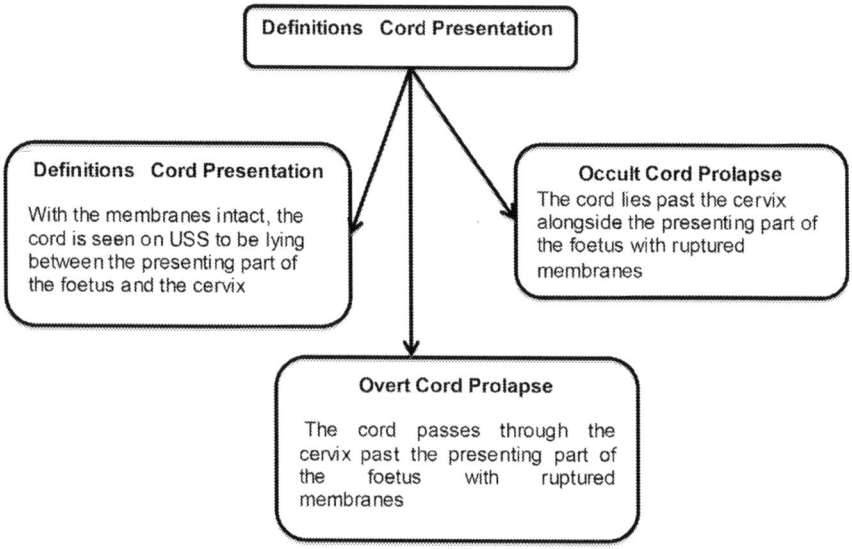

53.2 Cord prolapse management pathway

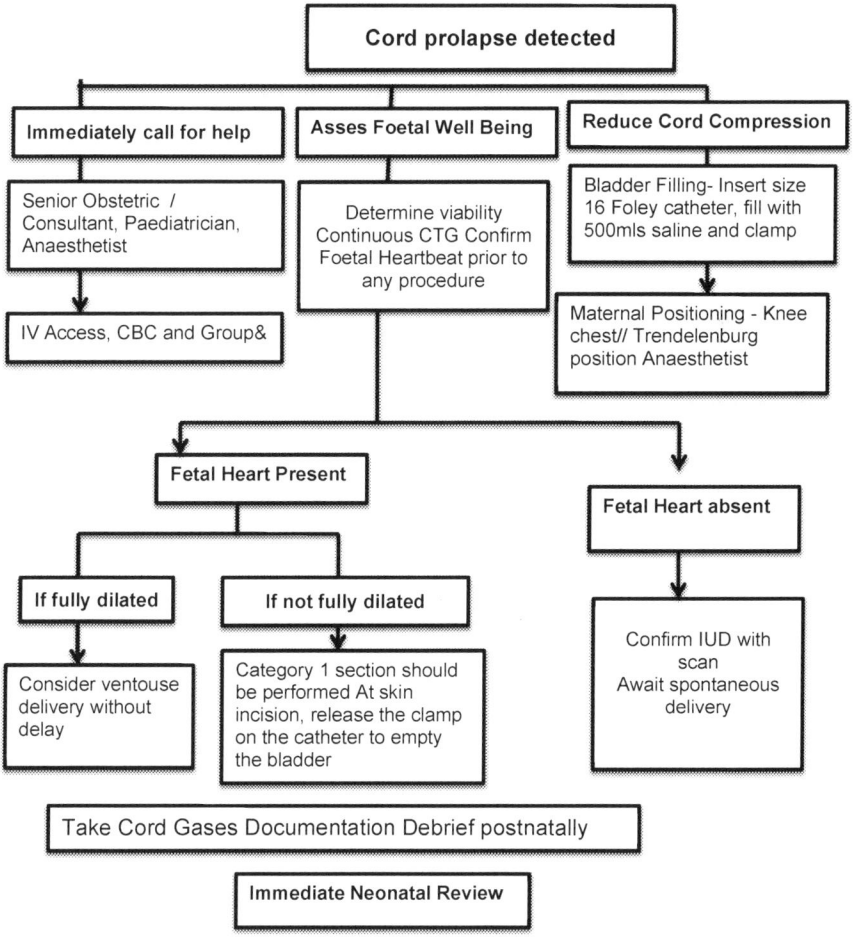

54 Uterine Inversion

54.1 Suspect uterine inversion

Suspect uterine inversion

Recognition

- Severe lower abdominal pain in 3rd Stage of labour
- Haemorrhage (94%)
- Shock that is out of proportion to blood loss owing to vagal stimulation
- Placenta may or may not be in place
- uterine fundus not palpable per abdomen
- Pelvic examination shows mass in the vagina or outside the introitus

54.2 Management of uterine inversion

Management of uterine inversion

Call for help from experienced obstetrician/ Anaesthetist/midwives

Stop Syntocinon if on flow

Take the anti shock measures

- Insert 2 wide bore cannula (14 to 16G)
- Collect blood for FBC, coagulation studies, group and cross match 4-6 units
- Start fluid replacements immediately (crystalloids)
- Monitor BP, pulse, urine output, O2 saturation continuously

↓

Transfer to theatre

After given appropriate analgesia

Consider tocolytics to facilitate replacement of uterus (MgS04 2-4g IV 5 mints)Terbutaline 0.25 mgm IV/Nitroglycerine 100 mgm IV

Attempt to reposition the uterus

-Manual replacement (Johnson maneuver)

-O'Sullivan's technique infuse 2-3 liters warm saline into posterior fornix of the vagina (use Ventouse silicon cup)

-Surgery - *Huntingdon's method **Houltains technique

-Oxytocin administered after repositioning (post replacement)/ -Do not remove placenta, leave until after repositioning / IV prophylactic antibiotics /-Thromboprophylaxis as per protocol

55 Ruptured uterus

55.1 Risk factors for uterine rupture

Risk factor

Obesity
• uterine scar
• Oxytocic in the multigravida woman or with previous caesarean scar
• Gran multiparty
• Diagnosed CPD
• Malpresentation
• Placenta accrete
• Macrosomic

Warning sign

Scar pain and tenderness
• Persistent pain between contractions
• Vaginal bleeding
• Fetal distress
• Fetal heart rate decelerati fetus
• Uterine abnormality
• Prior

55.2 Ruptured uterus management pathway

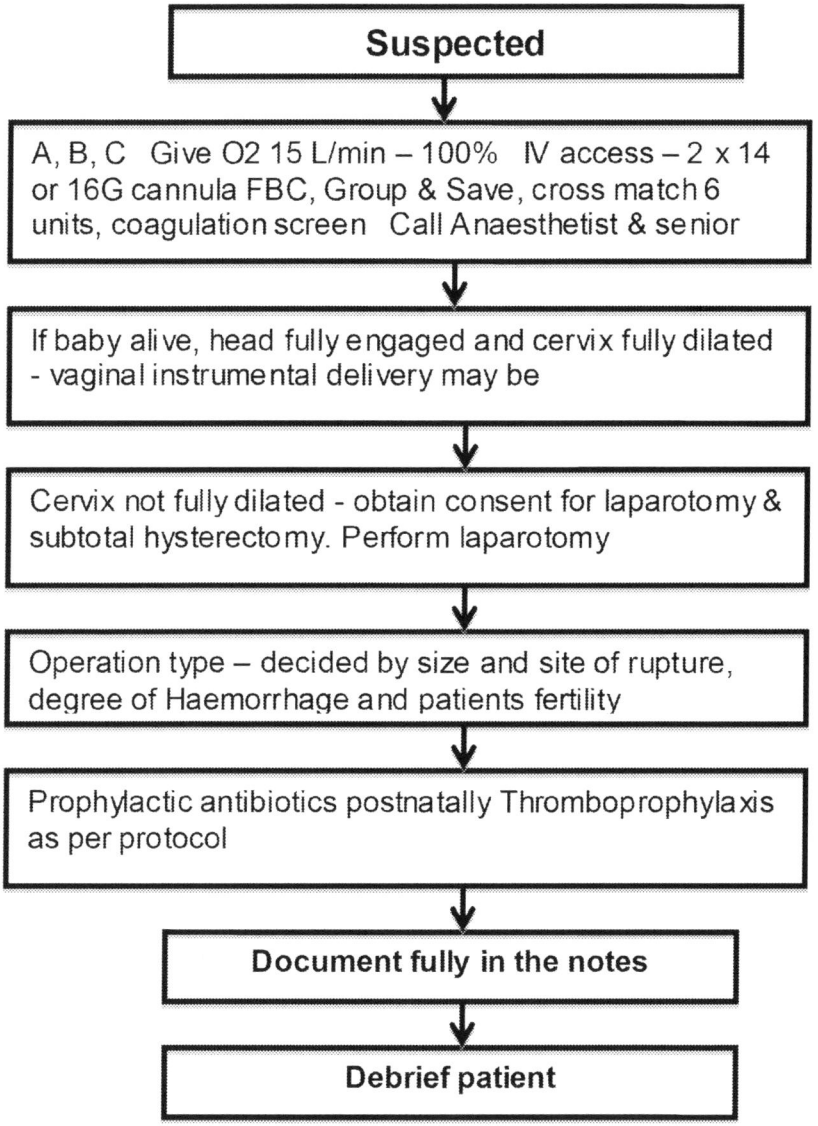

56 Retained Placenta

56.1 Definition

Definition: Placenta undelivered after 30mins

56.2 Retained placenta management

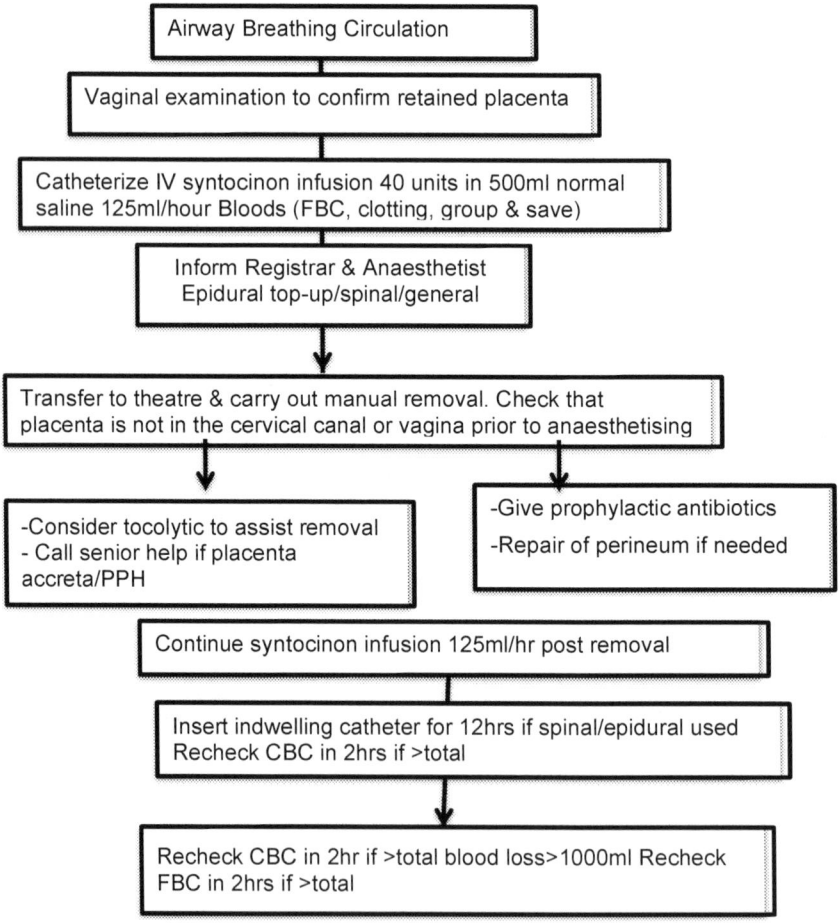

57 Care plan for women in labor if blood not available

IV access.

CBC, Group & Save.

Inform consultant obstetrician and Anaesthetist.

Active management of 3rd stage of labor.

Do not leave the patient alone for first hour after delivery.

IV Oxytocin infusion if any risk factors of PPH present.

57.1 Management Of Postpartum Anaemia

1.Severe anemia – involve hematologist. Give oxygen use recombinant human erythropoietin's 300 units/kg – three-weekly subcutaneously.

Augment with iron, vitamin B12 and folic acid.

2.IV Ferrous inject 1 gram if patient > 70 Kg- 15 minute infusion.

3.Consider elective ventilation in ICU.

4.Hyperbaric oxygen therapy – in life threatening anemia.
Contacts: Hospital Liaison Committee for Jehovah's Witnesses

57.2 Management in active hemorrhage in labor if blood not avialable

57.3 1st step in active hemorrhage management

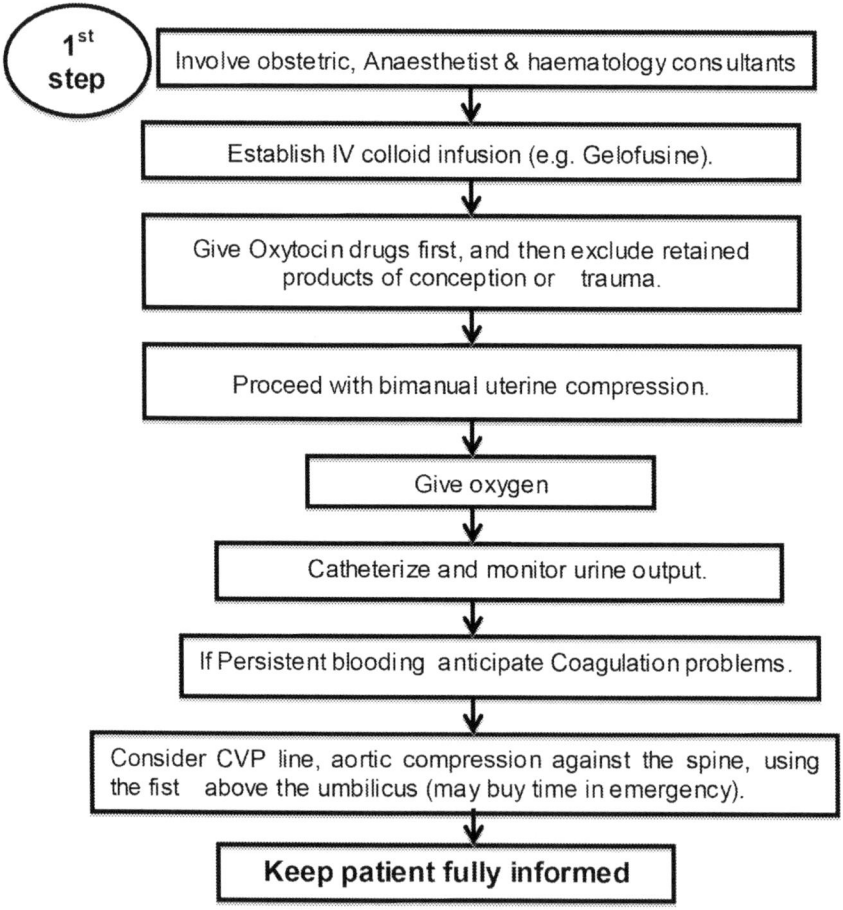

57.4 2nd step in active hemorrhage management pathway

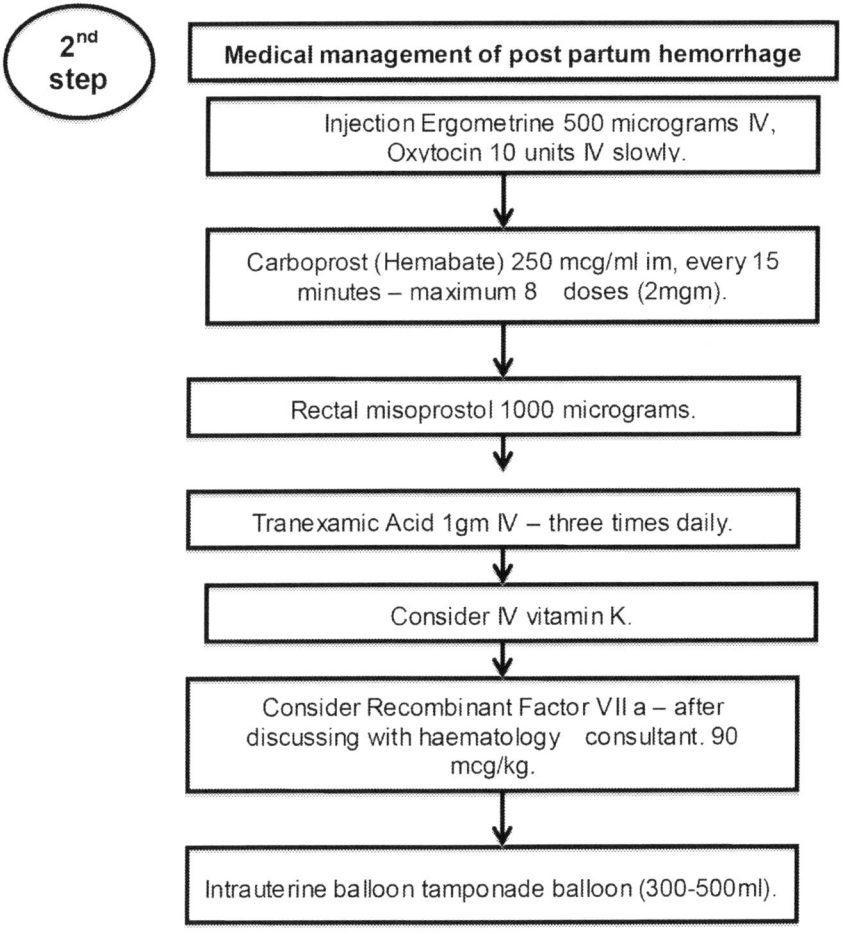

57.5 Surgical management of post partum hemorrhage pathway

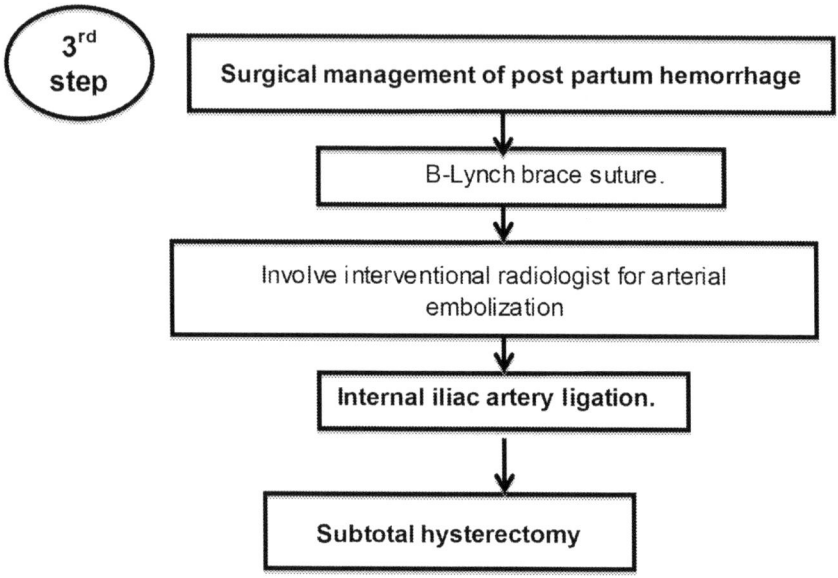

58 Management of Post Partum Hemorrhage

58.1 Risk Factors for Post Partum Hemorrhage

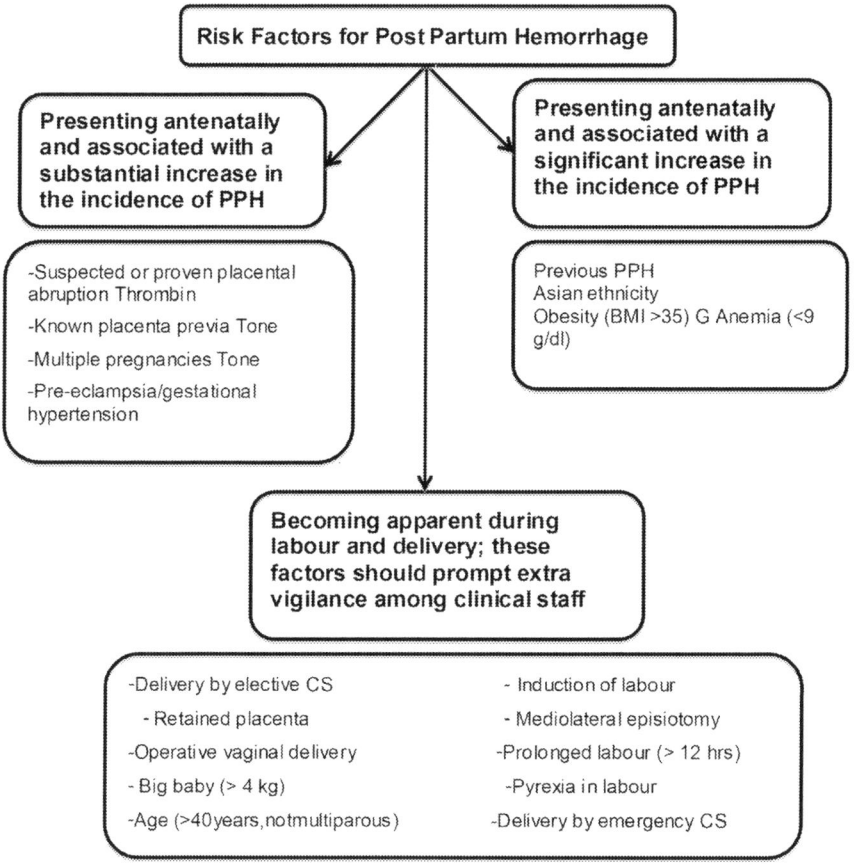

58.2 Definition& general measure to stabilize patient with PPH pathway

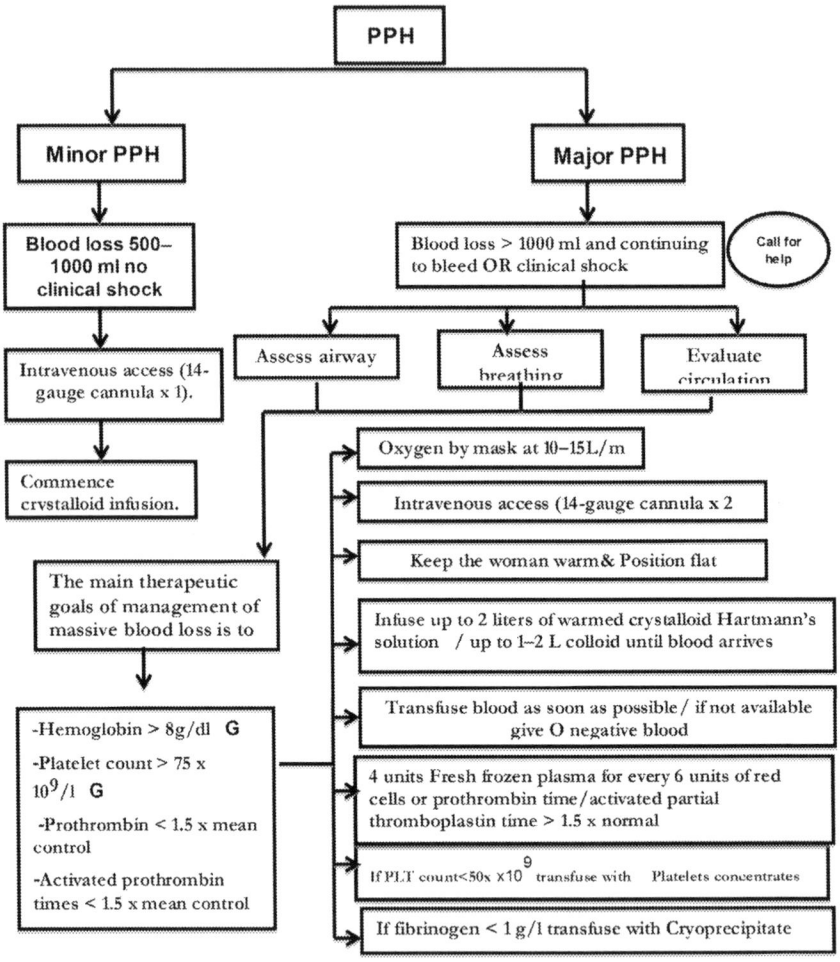

59 Massive transfusion

59.1 Management of patient with massive blood loss

Massive transfusion, defined as
The replacement by transfusion of more than 50 percent of a patient's blood volume in 12 to 24 hours,

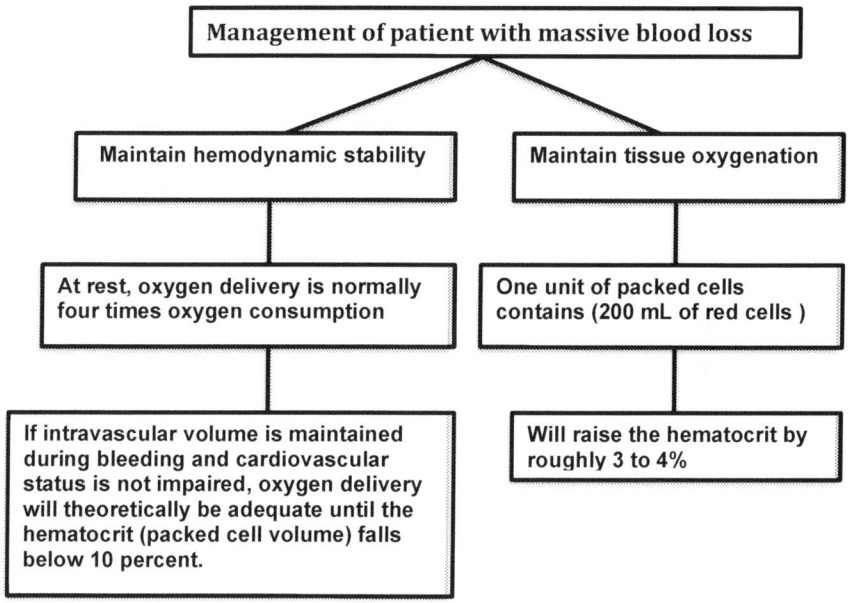

59.2 Treatment of patient with severe hypovolemia or hypovolemic shock

Treatment of patient with severe hypovolemia or hypovolemic shock

The principle of fluid resuscitation

The rate of fluid replacement

2-3 liters of isotonic saline are initially given as rapidly as possible in an attempt to restore tissue perfusion

Fluid repletion should continue at the initial rapid rate as long as the systemic blood pressure remains low. Clinical signs, including blood pressure, urine output, mental status, and peripheral perfusion, are often adequate to guide resuscitation.

A central venous catheter should be considered in patients who fail to respond to initial fluid resuscitation

The role for buffer therapy in patients with concurrent lactic acidosis

The type of fluid infused

Saline solutions are equally effective as colloid in expanding the plasma volume Colloid-containing solutions are not more effective in preserving pulmonary function

Starch solutions have been associated with coagulopathy, and increased risk of acute kidney injury

Lactated-Ringers solution or 0.45% saline solution with 75 mmol/L of sodium bicarbonate) be used instead of isotonic saline for large volume resuscitation.

Large volume resuscitation using isotonic saline may be associated with hyperchloremic metabolic acidosis &renal vasoconstriction and decreased glomerular filtration further disturbed electrolyte in ICU patient

Patients with marked hypo perfusion may develop lactic acidosis, leading to a reduction in extracellular pH below 7.10. Sodium bicarbonate has been added to the replacement fluid in this setting

59.3 Complication of massive blood transfusion

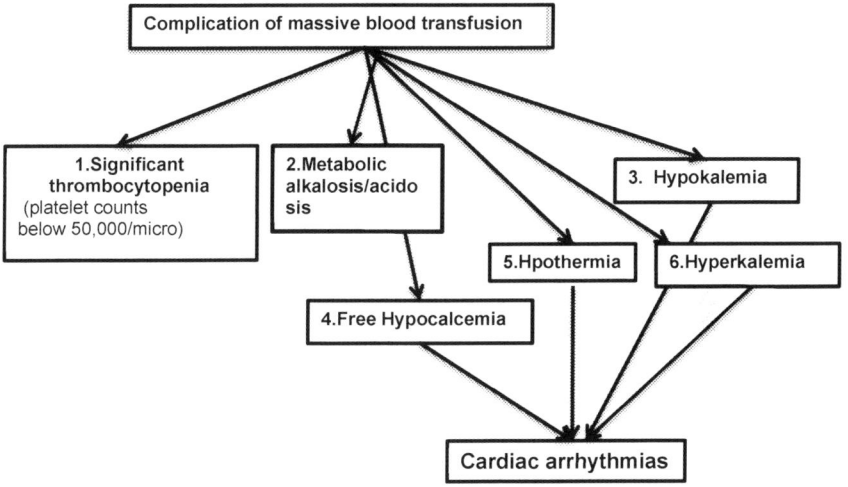

59.4 If the Patient require blood transfusion>5 unit

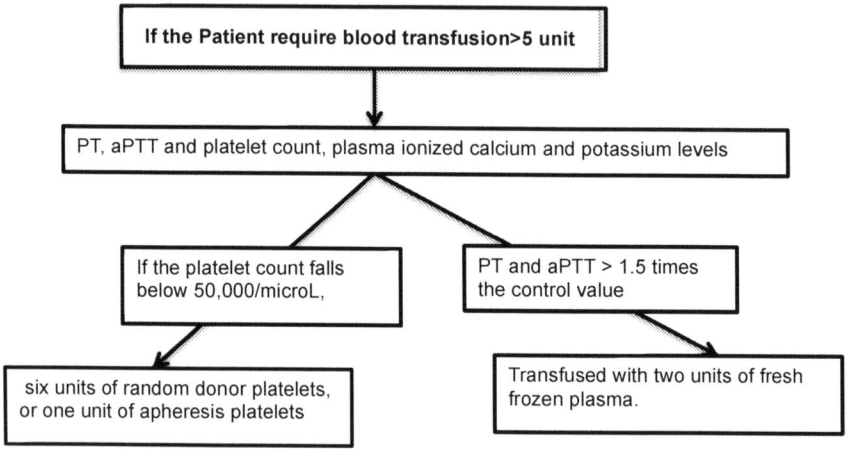

59.5 Complication of massive blood transfusion

Complication of massive blood transfusion

1.Significant thrombocytopenia
(platelet counts below 50,000/micro)

For each 10 to 12 units of transfused red cells can produce a 50 percent fall in the platelet count

One apheresis concentrate should increase the platelet count by 5000 to 10,000/microL

2.Metabolic alkalosis/acidosis

The pH of a unit of blood at the time of collection is 7.10 The pH then falls 0.1 pH unit/week due to the production of lactic and pyruvic acids by the red cells.

Citrate will generate a total of 23 meq of bicarbonate in each unit of blood

Maintain: Oxygenation, Cardiac output &Tissue perfusion

Metabolic alkalosis can occur if the renal ischemia or underlying renal disease prevents the excess bicarbonate from being excreted in the urine. This may be accompanied by hypokalemia as potassium moves into cells in exchange for hydrogen ions that move out of the cells to minimize the degree of extracellular alkalosis

3.Hypokalemia

Blood is anticoagulated with sodium citrate which increase the bicarbonate and this lead to metabolic alkalosis H+ shift from intracellular to extracellular ,k will shift to intracellular causing hypokalemia

4. Hypocalcemia

Citrate will combine with ionized calcium this will lead to significant fall in the plasma free calcium concentration and increase in Free hypocalcemia which lead to Paresthesias & cardiac arrhythmias treat hypocalcemia by10 %calcium gluconate give 10 to 20ml for every 500 mL of blood infused.

5.Hpothermia

Use fluid warmers, Remove wet linen, Provide warmer blankets and monitor temperature at least Q 15 minutes

6. Hyperkalemia

Patient with renal impairment may develop hyperkalemia because of potassium leakage due to prolonged blood storage or irradiation

To minimize the risk of hyperkalemia

1.Select only red cells collected less than five days prior to transfusion.2.Any unit of red cells can be washed immediately before infusion to remove extracellular potassium

Patients with severe massive blood replacement, and coagulopathy have improved survival when the ratio of transfused FFP (units) to transfused platelets (units) to red cells (units) approaches **1:1:1**

Laboratory

Base line investigation

CBC, coagulation profile (PT, APTT, fibrinogen), biochemistry (electrolytes and liver function tests, include Ca2+ and lactate), arterial blood gases (ABG)

Follow up investigation

CBC, coagulation profile (PT, APTT, fibrinogen), serum electrolytes include Ca2+ and lactate, (ABG)

Target Results

-pH greater than 7.20

-Base deficit greater than minus 6

-Lactate less than 4 mmol/L

-Ca2+ greater than 1.1 mmol/L

Platelets greater than 50 X 10^9/L

-PT and aPTT less than 1.5 x normal

-Fibrinogen greater than 2.5 g/L

59.6 Causes for PPH 'the four Ts'

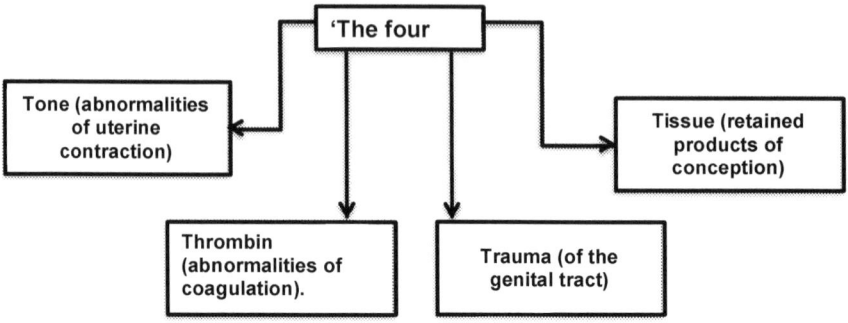

59.7 Medical Management of uterine atony pathway

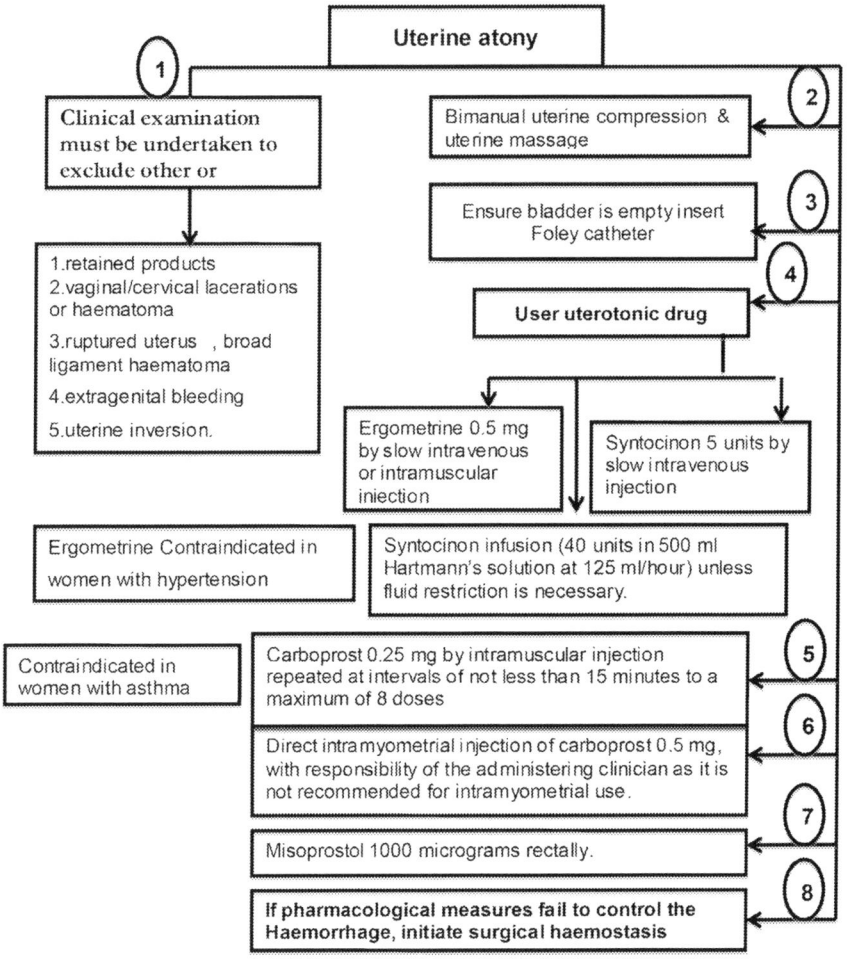

59.8 Surgical management of uterine atony pathway

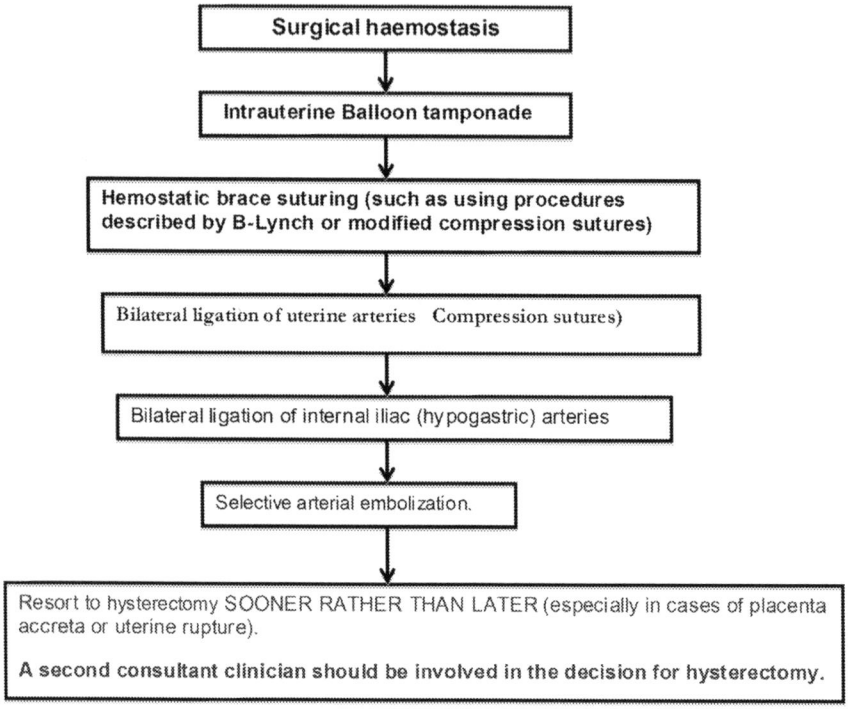

60 Intra-Partum Collapse

60.1 Uterine Rupture

Uterine Rupture

Note any previous history of uterine surgery, e.g. caesarean section, myomectomy, ectopic pregnancy

60.2 Eclampsia

Eclampsia

The women may be admitted from home fitted with no previous history of PIH.

60.3 Pulmonary Embolism Amniotic Fluid Embolism

Pulmonary Embolism Amniotic Fluid Embolism

Presentation of Amniotic Fluid Embolism

-Sudden dyspnea, hypoxia and hypotension, which may be followed in minutes by cardio-respiratory arrest.
- Grand mal seizures.
-In survival left ventricular failure may develop in clinical picture consistent with adult respiratory distress

Risk factors for amniotic embolus include

•High parity.
•Excessive or strong contractions.
•The use of oxytocin drugs, in particular a single Intravenous bolus dose of Syntocinon or Syntometrine.
•Over distension of the uterus, e.g. Polyhydramnios.
•Uterine rupture.

The diagnosis can only be confirmed after the event by finding evidence of fetal squamous cells and much in peripheral vasculature.
Blood should be taken during the acute event for this purpose especially if a Swan Ganz catheter is inserted.

60.4 Neurological Causes

Neurological Causes

Epilepsy
Intracranial haemorrhage
Cerebral infarction.

60.5 Cardiac causes.

Cardiac causes.

Known case of cardiac disease ,patient seen & evaluated by cardiologist

Condition that occure suddenly in labour room causing intrapartum colaps arrhythmia or myocardial infarction due to ischemic heart disease can present in pregnancy as can cardiomyopathy and rupture aortic aneurysm.

A chest X-ray and ECG should be considered in any women presenting with chest pain particularly is she has hypertension

60.6 Cardiac Arrest

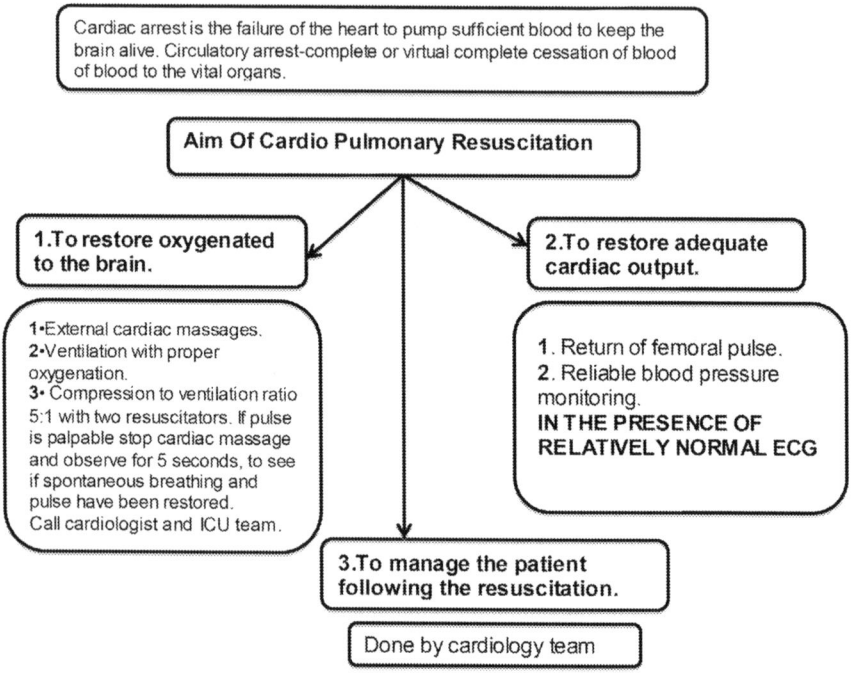

61 Management of delivery in cardiac disease patient

61.1 Aim and purpose

Aim and purpose

Timing and mode of delivery should be discussed in advance in a multidisciplinary team consisting of at least an obstetrician, an anesthesiologist, and a cardiologist.

The patient's should be thoroughly counseled about the delivery plan and potential complications.

A written record should be available at all times for all involved caregivers and should include plans to manage foreseeable complications.

61.2 Timing of delivery

Timing of delivery

Asymptomatic women in good condition	Wait for spontaneous labor
In women with complex lesions - Severe cardiac dysfunction - Heart failure - Aortic dilatation - Eisenmenger syndrome - Mechanical valve switched to heparin	Planned delivery might be more appropriate. Maternal or fetal condition might warrant a planned delivery before 37 weeks

61.3 Mode of delivery

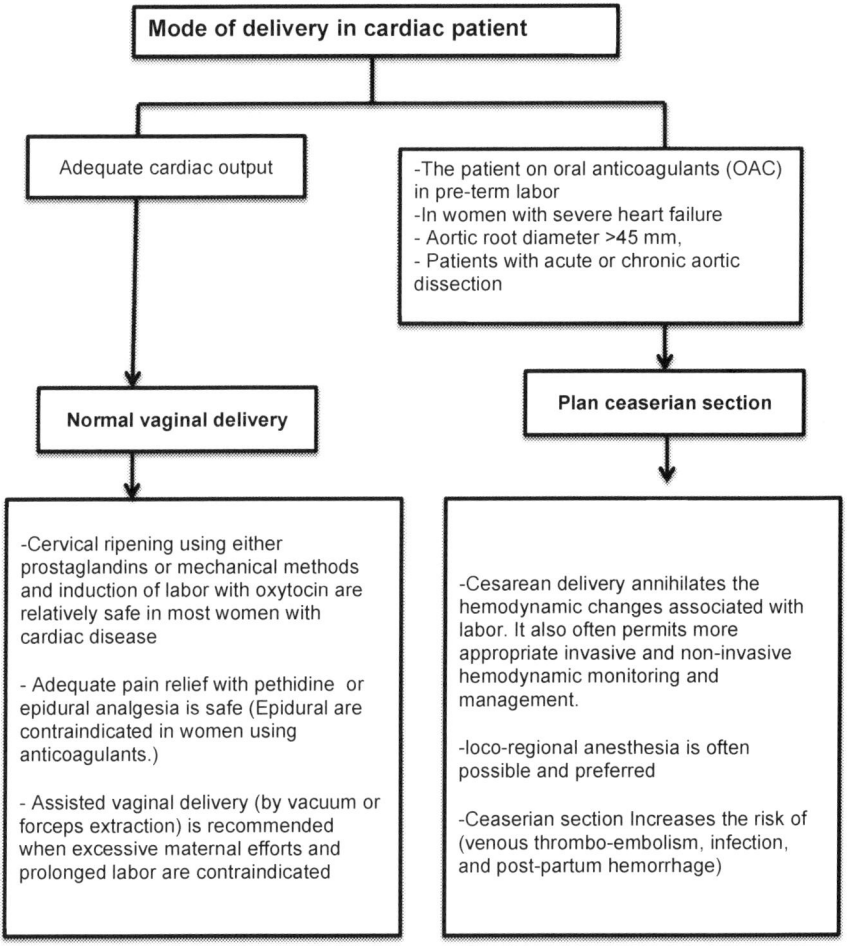

61.4 Prophylaxis antibiotics in cardiac patient

Prophylaxis antibiotics in cardiac patient

Preventive antibiotics are generally recommended for high risk patient with the following conditions

1.A prosthetic heart valve

2.Valve repair with prosthetic material

3.A prior history of Infected Endocarditis

4.Many congenital (from birth) heart abnormalities, such as single ventricle states, transposition of the great arteries, and tetralogy of Fallot, even if the abnormality has been repaired. Patent foramen ovale,

5. Pregnant women who are at highest risk for Infected Endocarditis should take an antibiotic before certain dental, oral, or upper respiratory tract procedures

A pregnant woman who has a high risk of Infected Endocarditis does NOT usually need antibiotic prophylaxis before a normal vaginal delivery or cesarean section. Antibiotics may be recommended before labor or cesarean section for other reasons, including prevention of complications related to group B Streptococcus.

61.5 Post-partum period in cardiac patient

Post-partum period in cardiac patient

-Manage the 3rd stage of labour by oxytocin intravenous infusion
-Intravenous bolus of oxytocine might cause a sudden fall in cardiac output
- Intravenous prostaglandins, can cause coronary vasospasms

Post-partum period in cardiac patient

High-risk patients

(Patients with diminished left ventricular function)Consider

-Several days of close monitoring for signs of heart failure is recommended.
- Prophylactic diuretics and ACE inhibitors may be indicated in high-risk patients.
- A routine echocardiographic examination post-delivery in high-risk women is advisable, paying careful attention to the aortic root in women with Marfan syndrome or aortic valve disease.
-The risk of thrombo-embolic complications is further increased post-partum and anticoagulation should be adjusted accordingly.

Low -risk patients

For heart failure and with normal ventricular function,

-a short observation period of several hours up to 48 h post-partum might be sufficient.

Lactation is possible in most women with heart disease; it might be contraindicated due to medication use, severely decreased effort tolerance, or risk of mastitis and bacteremia in some women. The use of diuretics can complicate the initiation of milk production.

62 Extremely Premature Babies between22and26weeks Gestation

62.1 Action in Established Pre-term Labour pathway

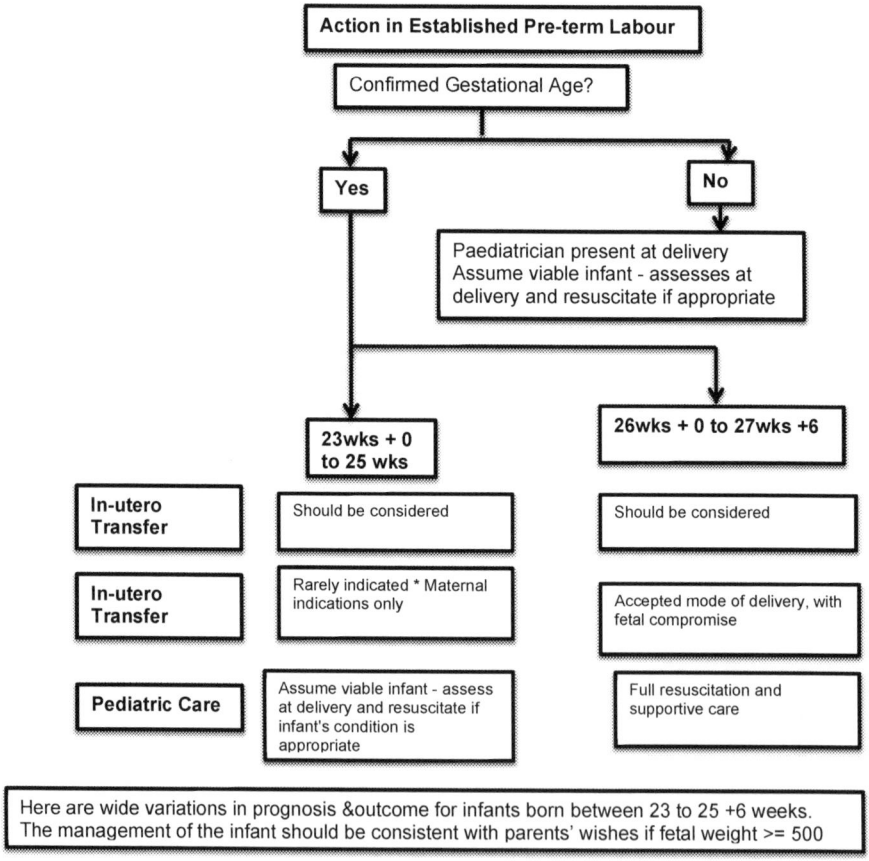

63 Late inter-uterine death and still birth

63.1 Definition

Definition

Delivery of a fetus with no signs of life known to have died after 24 completed weeks of gestation.

63.2 Diagnosis

Diagnosis

The diagnosis
-confirmed by ultrasound
-If patient wishes repeat USS should be offered by An appropriately trained person

Secondary features of IUD include
- Collapse of fetal skull and overlapping bones (Spalding's sign) - Maceration resulting in unrecognizable tissue
- Hydrops
- Intra foetal gas

Auscultation and CTG are unreliable an should not be used for diagnosis intra utrine fetal death

63.3 Communication

Communication

Parents should be told in the appropriate surroundings in an expert train person in breaking bad news .If alone, offer to call partner, family or friends Parents may need time to absorb any information

63.4 Isoimmunisation prevention

Isoimmunisation prevention

-Identify the patient blood group and Rh status

-if the patient Rh negative do Kleihauer testing

-administered anti D if needed within 72 hrs (can be given up to 10 days)

63.5 Mode of delivery and timing

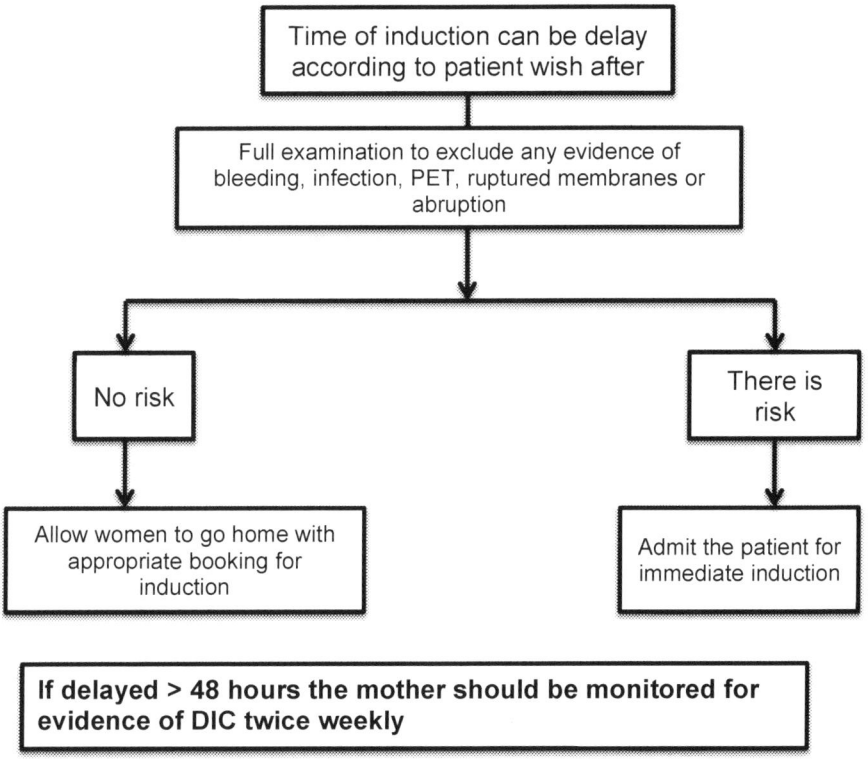

63.6 Mode of delivery

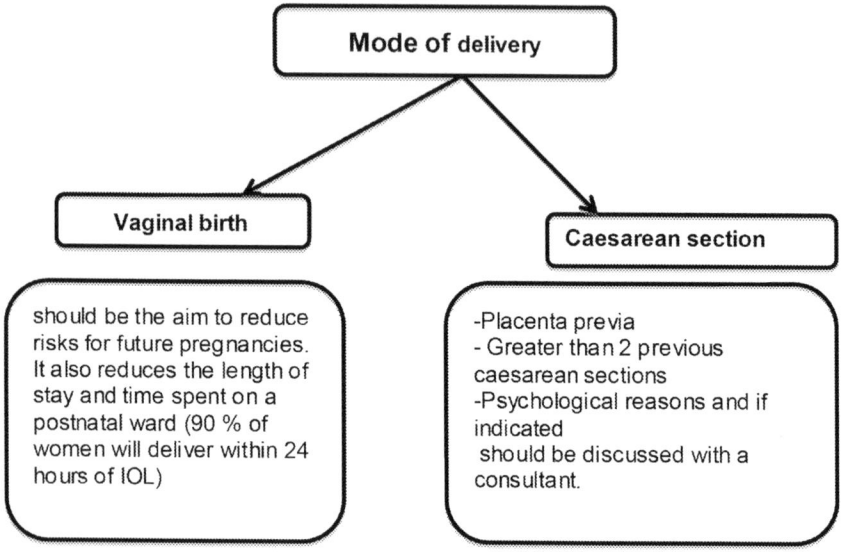

63.7 IOL see flowchart

IOL in IUFD

A combination of mifepristone and prostaglandin preparation should usually be recommended

Day 1: oral 200mg Mifepristone
Day 3: PV (break tablets in half) 100mcg 4hrly X 4 doses.

Prostaglandin induction
See the flow chart

-Syntocinon augmentation should be a consultant decision

-DO NOT rupture membranes to prevent chorioamnitis

-If previous uterine scar case discussed with consultant induction of labou according to flow chart
Women with 2 previous LSCS should be advised that in general the absolute risk of IOL with prostaglandin is only a little higher than for a women with single previous scar. Women with > 2 LSCS or atypical scars should be advised that the safety is unknown
Misoprostol can be used in preference to PG E2 due to its equivalent safety and efficiency with lower cost.

Antibiotics

Prophylaxis for GBS is not required if patient is known to be GBS
Antibiotics are not required unless there is evidence of infection

Thromboprophylaxis

Standard prophylaxis guidelines should be followed IUD is not a risk factor

Suppression of lactation

-Good breast support Ice packs NSAIDS
- Pharmacological suppression Cabergoline is superior to bromocriptine.
Cabergoline is an ergot derivative; it should not be used if there is a history of PET or a strong F/H of CVS disease or thromboembolic disease

1mg Carbergoline STAT during the first day post partum before lactation begins 250mcg 12 hourly for two days

if lactation has begun Bromocriptine (2.5mg BD) X 14 days.

63.8 Investigations

Investigations

Necessity of investigation should be explain th the cobbles . Following should be considered: CBC

-Kleihauer test Blood group and antibody screen

Coagulation and fibrinogen (abruption, DIC)

HbA1C if known diabetes, random blood glucose if not

Urea and Electrolytes Liver function tests Bile acids

TFT's (occult thyroid disease)

CRP, Blood cultures (sepsis)

Syphilis / Parvovirus / CMV / Toxoplasmosis / Rubella serology

Urine culture

High vaginal swab Cervical swabs Placental swab Placental histology

Fetal blood for culture Fetal skin swabs for culture Fetal skin biopsy / placental biopsy for karyotyping (NOT FIXED IN FORMALIN) Post mortem

64 Obstetric temple

64.1 Temple of vacuum delivery

64.2 Temple of forceps delivery

64.3 Temple of shoulder dystocia

Temple of vacuum delivery

Consent sign by patient

Name of obstetrician conducting the delivery ----------

title ----------

G-----P-------

PA head engagement --------- Fetal size ---------

Contraction ring yes no

Bladder evacuated yes no

Vaginal examination

Cervix ----------

Vertex station ----------

Patient on syntocinon yes no

Time h: m successful?

Application time: _____: _____

Traction start time: _____: _____

Delivery time: _____: _____

# of pulls: .....

Of pop-offs:----------

Time announce failed vacuum ---------

Delivery accomplished by:

__ Spontaneous vaginal delivery

__ Forceps (assisted vaginal delivery)

__ Cesarean delivery

Time for the baby delivery Baby A/S

Name of pediatrician attending the delivery

Title ----------

Time of call for pediatrician ----------

Time of arrival of pediatrician ----------

Baby umbilical arterial cord ph------ BD------co2------Hco3------

Baby umbilical venous cord ph------ BD------co2------Hco3------

Development of complication

Perineal laceration -------

3rd or 4th degree perineal tear ----------

Post partum Haemorrhage--------

Shoulder dystocia ----------

Any other complication ----------

Time of delivery of placenta ----------

Comment :

Was delivery vacuum extraction ?

Yes__ No__

If no, why?

__ Failure of descent

__Equipment failure

__ Fetal intolerance

__ Maternal intolerance

Temple of forceps delivery

Consent sign by patient

Name of obstetrician conducting the delivery ----------

title ----------

G------P-------

PA head engagement ---------- Fetal size ----------

Contraction ring yes no

Bladder evacuated yes no

Vaginal examination

Cervix ----------

Vertex station ----------

Patient on syntocinon yes no

Time h: m

Application time: _____: _____

Traction start time: _____: _____

Delivery time: _____: _____

# of pulls: _____

Delivery accomplished by

__ Spontaneous vaginal delivery

__ forceps delivery

__ Cesarean delivery

Time for the baby delivery Baby A/S

Name of pediatrician attending the delivery

Title ----------

Time of call for pediatrician ----------

Time of arrival of pediatrician ----------

Baby umbilical arterial cord ph------ BD-------co2-------Hco3------

Baby umbilical venous cord ph------ BD-------co2-------Hco3------

Development of complication

Perineal laceration ------

3rd or 4th degree perineal tear ----------

Post partum Haemorrhage----------

Shoulder dystocia ----------

Any other complication ----------

Time of delivery of placenta ----------

Comment

Application

Easy__ Moderate__ Difficult __

Rotation:

N/A __ Easy __ Moderate __ Difficult__

Traction

Easy __ Moderate __ Difficult__

Temple of shoulder dystocia

Name of midwife conducting the delivery ----------

Name of obstetrician conducting the delivery

title ----------

G-----P--------

PA head engagement ---------- Fetal size ----------

Shoulder dystocia anticipated yes no

Bladder evacuated yes no

Vaginal examination

Cervix ----------

Vertex station ----------

Patient on syntocinon yes no

Time of announce call for help

Time for arrival of obstetrician --------

Name of obstetrician

Title ----------

Time for the **MCROBERT's** maneuver

Time for the Anterior shoulder disimpaction

Time for the Wood Screw manoeuver

Time for deliver by posterior arm

Time for proceeds for Deliver posterior arm delivery

Proceeded for ceaserian section Zavenelli/symphisiotomy/cleidotomy

Time for the baby delivery

Baby A/S

Name of pediatrician attending the delivery

Title ----------

Time of call for pediatrician ----------

Time of arrival of pediatrician ----------

Baby umbilical arterial cord ph----- BD-------co2------Hco3-----

Baby umbilical venous cord ph------ BD-------co2-----Hco3------

Development of complication

Perineal laceration ----------

3rd or 4th degree perineal tear ----------

Post partum Haemorrhage---------

Neurological defecate ----------

Any other complication ----------

Time of delivery of placenta ----------

Comment

65 Reference

65.1 chapter 1 reference

1. NICE 2008Antenatal care for uncomplicated pregnancies Clinical guideline Published: 26 March 2008 Nice.org.uk/guidance/cg62
2. World Health Organization 2016 WHO recommendations on antenatal care for a positive pregnancy experience. I.World Health Organization.

65.2 chapter 2 reference

1. Deaton JL, Honoré GM, Huffman CS, Bauguess P. Early transvaginal ultrasound following an accurately dated pregnancy: the importance of finding a yolk sac or fetal heart motion. Hum Reprod 1997; 12:2820.
2. Nybo Andersen AM, Wohlfahrt J, Christens P, et al. Maternal age and fetal loss: population based register linkage study. BMJ 2000; 320:1708.
3. Savaris RF, de Moraes GS, Cristovam RA, Braun RD. Are antibiotics necessary after 48 hours of improvement in infected/septic abortions? A randomized controlled trial followed by a cohort study. Am J Obstet Gynecol 2011; 204:301.e1.
4. Sawaya GF, Grady D, Kerlikowske K, Grimes DA. Antibiotics at the time of induced abortion: the case for universal prophylaxis based on a meta-analysis. Obstet Gynecol 1996; 87:884.
5. Grossman D, Blanchard K, Blumenthal P. Complications after second trimester surgical and medical abortion. Reprod Health Matters 2008; 16:173.

65.3 chapter 3 referance

Reference

1. Boehlen F, Hohlfeld P, Extermann P, et al. Platelet count at term pregnancy: a reappraisal of the threshold. Obstet Gynecol 2000; 95:29.
2. Neunert C, Lim W, Crowther M, et al. The American Society of Hematology 2011 evidence-based practice guideline for immune thrombocytopenia. Blood 2011; 117:4190.
3. Gill KK, Kelton JG. Management of idiopathic thrombocytopenic purpura in pregnancy. Semin Hematol 2000; 37:275.
4. Webert KE, Mittal R, Sigouin C, et al. A retrospective 11-year analysis of obstetric patients with idiopathic thrombocytopenic purpura. Blood 2003; 102:4306.
5. Chong BH. Primary immune thrombocytopenia: understanding pathogenesis is the key to better treatments. J Thromb Haemost 2009; 7:319
6. Koyama S, Tomimatsu T, Kanagawa T, et al. Reliable predictors of neonatal immune thrombocytopenia in pregnant women with idiopathic thrombocytopenic purpura. Am J Hematol 2012; 87:15.
7. Allford SL, Hunt BJ, Rose P, et al. Guidelines on the diagnosis and management of the thrombotic microangiopathic haemolytic anaemias. Br J Haematol 2003; 120:556.
8. McMinn JR, George JN. Evaluation of women with clinically suspected thrombotic thrombocytopenic purpura-hemolytic uremic syndrome during pregnancy. J Clin Apher 2001; 16:202.
9. Webert KE, Mittal R, Sigouin C, et al. A retrospective 11-year analysis of obstetric patients with idiopathic thrombocytopenic purpura. Blood 2003; 102:4306.

65.4 Chapter 4 reference

1. Stephansson O, Dickman PW, Johansson A, Cnattingius S. Maternal hemoglobin concentration during pregnancy and risk of stillbirth. JAMA 2000; 284:2611.
2. Juncà J, Fernández-Avilés F, Oriol A, et al. The usefulness of the serum transferrin receptor in detecting iron deficiency in the anemia of chronic disorders. Haematologica 1998; 83:676.
3. Recommendations to prevent and control iron deficiency in the United States. Centers for Disease Control and Prevention. MMWR Morb Mortal Wkly Rep 1998; 47(RR-3):1.
4. Brugnara C. Iron deficiency and erythropoiesis: new diagnostic approaches. Clin Chem 2003; 49:1573.

65.5 Chapter 5 Reference

1. Moore TR. Amniotic fluid dynamics reflect fetal and maternal health and disease. Obstet Gynecol 2010; 116:759.
2. Zhu X, Jiang S, Hu Y, et al. The expression of aquaporin 8 and aquaporin 9 in fetal membranes and placenta in term pregnancies complicated by idiopathic polyhydramnios. Early Hum Dev 2010;
   86:657

65.6 Chapter 6 Reference

1. Moore TR. Amniotic fluid dynamics reflect fetal and maternal health and disease. Obstet Gynecol 2010; 116:759.
2. Zhu X, Jiang S, Hu Y, et al. The expression of aquaporin 8 and aquaporin 9 in fetal membranes and placenta in term pregnancies complicated by idiopathic polyhydramnios. Early Hum Dev 2010;
   86:657

65.7 chapter 7 Reference

1. Bahado-Singh RO, Kovanci E, Jeffres A, et al. The Doppler cerebroplacental ratio and perinatal outcome in intrauterine growth restriction. Am J Obstet Gynecol 1999; 180:750.
2. Chambers SE, Hoskins PR, Haddad NG, et al. A comparison of fetal abdominal circumference measurements and Doppler ultrasound in the prediction of small-for-dates babies and fetal compromise. Br J Obstet Gynaecol 1989; 96:803.
3. Ferrazzi E, Nicolini U, Kustermann A, Pardi G. Routine obstetric ultrasound: effectiveness of cross-sectional screening for fetal growth retardation. J Clin Ultrasound 1986; 14:17.
4. Zhang J, Mikolajczyk R, Grewal J, et al. Prenatal application of the individualized fetal growth reference. Am J Epidemiol 2011; 173:539.
5. Dugoff L, Lynch AM, Cioffi-Ragan D, et al. First trimester uterine artery Doppler abnormalities predict subsequent intrauterine growth restriction. Am J Obstet Gynecol 2005; 193:1208.
6. Vasconcelos RP, Brazil Frota Aragão JR, Costa Carvalho FH, et al. Differences in neonatal outcome in fetuses with absent versus reverse end-diastolic flow in umbilical artery Doppler. Fetal Diagn Ther 2010; 28:160.
7. Nozaki AM, Francisco RP, Fonseca ES, et al. Fetal hemodynamic changes following maternal betamethasone administration in pregnancies with fetal growth restriction and absent end-diastolic flow in the umbilical artery. Acta Obstet Gynecol Scand 2009; 88:350.

65.8 Chapter 8 Reference

1. Delzell JE Jr, Lefevre ML. Urinary tract infections during pregnancy. Am Fam Physician 2000; 61:713.
2. Nicolle LE, Bradley S, Colgan R, et al. Infectious Diseases Society of America guidelines for the diagnosis and treatment of asymptomatic bacteriuria in adults. Clin Infect Dis 2005; 40:643.
3. Lin K, Fajardo K, U.S. Preventive Services Task Force. Screening for asymptomatic bacteriuria in adults: evidence for the U.S. Preventive Services Task Force reaffirmation recommendation statement. Ann Intern Med 2008; 149:W20.
4. Schito GC, Naber KG, Botto H, et al. The ARESC study: an international survey on the antimicrobial resistance of pathogens involved in uncomplicated urinary tract infections. Int J Antimicrob Agents 2009; 34:407.
5. Archabald KL, Friedman A, Raker CA, Anderson BL. Impact of trimester on morbidity of acute pyelonephritis in pregnancy. Am J Obstet Gynecol 2009; 201:406.e1.

65.9 Chapter 9 Reference

1. Gonzalez MC, Reyes H, Arrese M, et al. Intrahepatic cholestasis of pregnancy in twin pregnancies. J Hepatol 1989; 9:84.
2. Bacq Y, Sapey T, Bréchot MC, et al. Intrahepatic cholestasis of pregnancy: a French prospective study. Hepatology 1997; 26:358.
3. Pusl T, Beuers U. Intrahepatic cholestasis of pregnancy. Orphanet J Rare Dis 2007; 2:26.
4. Williamson C, Hems LM, Goulis DG, et al. Clinical outcome in a series of cases of obstetric cholestasis identified via a patient support group. BJOG 2004; 111:676.

5. Glantz A, Marschall HU, Mattsson LA. Intrahepatic cholestasis of pregnancy: relationships between bile acid levels and fetal complication rates. Hepatology 2004;40:467–74.

65.10 Chapter 10

1. Lamont RF, Sobel JD, Carrington D, et al. Varicella-zoster virus (chickenpox) infection in pregnancy. BJOG 2011; 118:1155.
2. Cohen A, Moschopoulos P, Maschopoulos P, et al. Congenital varicella syndrome: the evidence for secondary prevention with varicella-zoster immune globulin. CMAJ 2011; 183:204.
3. Harger JH, Ernest JM, Thurnau GR, et al. Risk factors and outcome of varicella-zoster virus pneumonia in pregnant women. J Infect Dis 2002; 185:422.
4. Centers for Disease Control and Prevention (CDC). FDA approval of an extended period for administering VariZIG for postexposure prophylaxis of varicella. MMWR Morb Mortal Wkly Rep 2012; 61:212.

65.11 Chapter 11 Reference

1. Bahia-Oliveira LM, Jones JL, Azevedo-Silva J, et al. Highly endemic, waterborne toxoplasmosis in north Rio de Janeiro state, Brazil. Emerg Infect Dis 2003; 9:55.
2. Gilbert RE, Freeman K, Lago EG, et al. Ocular sequelae of congenital toxoplasmosis in Brazil compared with Europe. PLoS Negl Trop Dis 2008; 2:e277.
3. Binquet C, Wallon M, Quantin C, et al. [Evaluation of prevention strategies for congenital toxoplasmosis: a critical

review of medico-economic studies]. Rev Epidemiol Sante Publique 2002; 50:475.
4. Gilbert RE, Gras L, Wallon M, et al. Effect of prenatal treatment on mother to child transmission of Toxoplasma gondii: retrospective cohort study of 554 mother-child pairs in Lyon, France. Int J Epidemiol 2001; 30:1303.
5. Flack NJ, Sepulveda W, Bower S, Fisk NM. Acute maternal hydration in third-trimester oligohydramnios: effects on amniotic fluid volume, uteroplacental perfusion, and fetal blood flow and urine output. Am J Obstet Gynecol 1995; 173:1186.
6. Brace RA. Physiology of amniotic fluid volume regulation. Clin Obstet Gynecol 1997; 40:280.
7. Magann EF, Chauhan SP, Doherty DA, et al. A review of idiopathic hydramnios and pregnancy outcomes. Obstet Gynecol Surv 2007; 62:795.
8. Kramer MS, Rouleau J, Baskett TF, et al. Amniotic-fluid embolism and medical induction of labour: a retrospective, population-based cohort study. Lancet2006; 368:1444.

65.12 Chapter 12 Reference

1. Centers for Disease Control and Prevention (CDC). Cephalosporin susceptibility among Neisseria gonorrhoeae isolates--United States, 2000-2010. MMWR Morb Mortal Wkly Rep 2011; 60:873.
2. file://www.cdc.gov/std/treatment/2010/default.htm (Accessed on January 13, 2011)
3. Centers for Disease Control and Prevention (CDC). Update to CDC's Sexually transmitted diseases treatment guidelines, 2010: oral cephalosporins no longer a recommended treatment for gonococcal infections. MMWR Morb Mortal Wkly Rep 2012; 61:590.

65.13 Chapter 13 Reference

1. Sookoian S. Liver disease during pregnancy: acute viral hepatitis. Ann Hepatol 2006; 5:231.
2. Tan HH, Lui HF, Chow WC. Chronic hepatitis B virus (HBV) infection in pregnancy. Hepatol Int 2008; 2:370.
3. Gill US, et al. Factors determining bone mineral density loss in chronic hepatitis B patients: is tenofovir disoproxil fumarate the main culprit? Gut 2011; 60:A230.
4. Hill JB, Sheffield JS, Kim MJ, et al. Risk of hepatitis B transmission in breast-fed infants of chronic hepatitis B carriers. Obstet Gynecol 2002; 99:1049.

65.14 Chapter 14 Reference

1. Stagno, S. Britt, W. Cytomegalovirus infections. In: Infectious Diseases of the Fetus and Newborn Infant, 6th ed, Remington, JS, Klein, JO, Wilson, CB, Baker, CJ (Eds), Elsevier Saunders, Philadelphia 2006. p.739.
2. Ross SA, Novak Z, Pati S, et al. Mixed infection and strain diversity in congenital cytomegalovirus infection. J Infect Dis 2011; 204:1003.
3. Simonazzi G, Guerra B, Bonasoni P, et al. Fetal cerebral periventricular halo at midgestation: an ultrasound finding suggestive of fetal cytomegalovirus infection. Am J Obstet Gynecol 2010; 202:599.e1.
4. Lipitz S, Hoffmann C, Feldman B, et al. Value of prenatal ultrasound and magnetic resonance imaging in assessment of congenital primary cytomegalovirus infection. Ultrasound Obstet Gynecol 2010; 36:709.

65.15 Chapter 15 Reference:

1. Management of genital Herpes in Pregnancy, RCOG Green-top guideline No. 30, September 2007
2. Baker DA. Management of Herpes in Pregnancy. ACOG Practice Bulletin 8. Washington, DC: American College of Obstetricians and Gynecologists, 1999.
3. Brown ZA, Wald A, Morrow RA, Selke S, Zeh J, Corey L. Effect of serologic status and cesarean delivery on transmission rate of herpes simplex virus from mother to infant. JAMA 2003;289:203–9.

65.16 Chapter 16 Reference

1. Miyagawa S, Takahashi Y, Nagai A, et al. Angio-oedema in a neonate with IgG antibodies to parvovirus B19 following intrauterine parvovirus B19 infection. Br J Dermatol 2000; 143:428.
2. Prospective study of human parvovirus (B19) infection in pregnancy. Public Health Laboratory Service Working Party on Fifth Disease. BMJ 1990; 300:1166.
3. Enders M, Weidner A, Rosenthal T, et al. Improved diagnosis of gestational parvovirus B19 infection at the time of nonimmune fetal hydrops. J Infect Dis 2008; 197:58.
4. Borna S, Mirzaie F, Hanthoush-Zadeh S, et al. Middle cerebral artery peak systolic velocity and ductus venosus velocity in the investigation of nonimmune hydrops. J Clin Ultrasound 2009; 37:385.

65.17 Chapter 17 reference

1. Rodis JF, Quinn DL, Gary GW Jr, et al. Management and outcomes of pregnancies complicated by human B19

parvovirus infection: a prospective study. Am J Obstet Gynecol 1990; 163:1168.
2. Skjöldebrand-Sparre L, Tolfvenstam T, Papadogiannakis N, et al. Parvovirus B19 infection: association with third-trimester intrauterine fetal death. BJOG 2000; 107:476.
3. Marton T, Martin WL, Whittle MJ. Hydrops fetalis and neonatal death from human parvovirus B19: an unusual complication. Prenat Diagn 2005; 25:543.
4. Cosmi E, Mari G, Delle Chiaie L, et al. Noninvasive diagnosis by Doppler ultrasonography of fetal anemia resulting from parvovirus infection. Am J Obstet Gynecol 2002; 187:1290.

65.18 Chapter 18 Referance

1. FIUMARA NJ. Congenital syphilis in Massachusetts. N Engl J Med 1951; 245:634.
2. Centers for Disease Control and Prevention (CDC). Congenital syphilis - United States, 2003-2008. MMWR Morb Mortal Wkly Rep 2010; 59:413.
3. U.S. Preventive Services Task Force. Screening for syphilis infection in pregnancy: U.S. Preventive Services Task Force reaffirmation recommendation statement. Ann Intern Med 2009; 150:705.
4. American College of Obstetricians and Gynecologists and American Academy of Pediatrics. Guidelines for Perinatal Care, 7th edition, 2012.
5. Yates AB. Management of patients with a history of allergy to beta-lactam antibiotics. Am J Med 2008; 121:572.

65.19 Chapter 19 Reference

1. Phylipsen M, Yamsri S, Treffers EE, et al. Non-invasive prenatal diagnosis of beta-thalassemia and sickle-cell

disease using pyrophosphorolysis-activated polymerization and melting curve analysis. Prenat Diagn 2012; 32:578.
2. Wang X, Seaman C, Paik M, et al. Experience with 500 prenatal diagnoses of sickle cell diseases: the effect of gestational age on affected pregnancy outcome. Prenat Diagn 1994; 14:851.
3. Martin JN Jr, Martin RW, Morrison JC. Acute management of sickle cell crisis in pregnancy. Clin Perinatol 1986; 13:853.
4. Jans SM, de Jonge A, Lagro-Janssen AL. Maternal and perinatal outcomes amongst haemoglobinopathy carriers: a systematic review. Int J Clin Pract 2010; 64:1688.
5. Winder AD, Johnson S, Murphy J, Ehsanipoor RM. Epidural analgesia for treatment of a sickle cell crisis during pregnancy. Obstet Gynecol 2011; 118:495.

65.20 Chapter 20 Reference

1. Yamazaki K, Sato K, Shizume K, et al. Potent thyrotropic activity of human chorionic gonadotropin variants in terms of 125I incorporation and de novo synthesized thyroid hormone release in human thyroid follicles. J Clin Endocrinol Metab 1995; 80:473.
2. Bajoria R, Fisk NM. Permeability of human placenta and fetal membranes to thyrotropin-stimulating hormone in vitro. Pediatr Res 1998; 43:621.
3. Stagnaro-Green A, Abalovich M, Alexander E, et al. Guidelines of the American Thyroid Association for the diagnosis and management of thyroid disease during pregnancy and postpartum. Thyroid 2011; 21:1081.
4. Idris I, Srinivasan R, Simm A, Page RC. Maternal hypothyroidism in early and late gestation: effects on neonatal and obstetric outcome. Clin Endocrinol (Oxf) 2005; 63:560.

5. hangaratinam S, Tan A, Knox E, et al. Association between thyroid autoantibodies and miscarriage and preterm birth: meta-analysis of evidence. BMJ 2011; 342:d2616.
6. Azizi F, Khoshniat M, Bahrainian M, Hedayati M. Thyroid function and intellectual development of infants nursed by mothers taking methimazole. J Clin Endocrinol Metab 2000; 85:3233.
7. Huel C, Guibourdenche J, Vuillard E, et al. Use of ultrasound to distinguish between fetal hyperthyroidism and hypothyroidism on discovery of a goiter. Ultrasound Obstet Gynecol 2009; 33:412.

65.21 Chapter 21 Reference

1. Metzger BE, Coustan DR (Eds.): Proceed- ings of the Fourth International Work- shop-Conference on Gestational Diabetes Mellitus. Diabetes Care 21 (Suppl. 2):B1– B167, 1998
2. International Association of Diabetes and Pregnancy Study Groups Consensus Panel, Metzger BE, Gabbe SG, Persson B, Buchanan TA, Catalano PA, Damm P, et al. International association of diabetes and pregnancy study groups recommendations on the diagnosis and classification of hyperglycemia in pregnancy. Diabetes Care 2010;33:676–82.
3. Kim C, Liu T, Valdez R, Beckles GL. Does frank diabetes in first-degree relatives of a pregnant woman affect the likelihood of her developing gestational diabetes mellitus or nongestational diabetes? Am J Obstet Gynecol 2009; 201:576.e1.
4. Lowe LP, Metzger BE, Dyer AR, et al. Hyperglycemia and Adverse Pregnancy Outcome (HAPO) Study: associations of maternal A1C and glucose with pregnancy outcomes. Diabetes Care 2012; 35:574.

5. 30. Landon MB, Mele L, Spong CY, et al. The relationship between maternal glycemia and perinatal outcome. Obstet Gynecol 2011; 117:218.
6. 10. Han S, Crowther, CA, et al. Different types of dietary advice for women with gestational diabetes mellitus. Cochrane Database Syst Rev 2013; :CD009275.
7. Metzger BE, Ravnikar V, Vileisis RA, Freinkel N. "Accelerated starvation" and the skipped breakfast in late normal pregnancy. Lancet 1982; 1:588.
8. Rizzo T, Metzger BE, Burns WJ, Burns K. Correlations between antepartum maternal metabolism and child intelligence. N Engl J Med 1991; 325:911.

65.22 Chapter 22 Reference

1. Wier LM, Witt E, Burgess J, Elixhauser A. A Healthcare Cost and Utilization Project. Statistical Brief 102. Hospitalizations Related to Diabetes in Pregnancy 2008, Agency for Health Care Policy and Research, Rockville, MD. 2010.
2. Ehrlich SF, Crites YM, Hedderson MM, et al. The risk of large for gestational age across increasing categories of pregnancy glycemia. Am J Obstet Gynecol 2011; 204:240. e1.
3. Holmes VA, Young IS, Patterson CC, et al. Optimal glycemic control, pre-eclampsia, and gestational hypertension in women with type 1 diabetes in the diabetes and pre-eclampsia intervention trial. Diabetes Care 2011; 34:1683.
4. NICE 2015.

65.23 Chapter 23 Reference

1. Sibai BM. Chronic hypertension in pregnancy. Obstet Gynecol 2002; 100:369–77.

2. Executive summary: hypertension in pregnancy. American Col- lege of Obstetricians and Gynecologists. Obstet Gynecol 2013; 122:1122–31.
3. Bujold E, Roberge S, Lacasse Y et al. (2010) Prevention of preeclampsia and intrauterine growth restriction with aspirin started in early pregnancy. Obstetrics & Gynecology 116: 402–12 abstract: www.greenjournal/Abstract/2010/08000
4. Hypertension in pregnancy: Evidence update May2012

65.24 Chapter 25 Reference

1. Mintz G, Niz J, Gutierrez G, et al. Prospective study of pregnancy in systemic lupus erythematosus. Results of a multidisciplinary approach. J Rheumatol 1986; 13:732.
2. Ruiz-Irastorza G, Khamashta MA. Lupus and pregnancy: ten questions and some answers. Lupus 2008; 17:416.
3. Kong NC. Pregnancy of a lupus patient--a challenge to the nephrologist. Nephrol Dial Transplant 2006; 21:268.
4. Chakravarty EF, Colón I, Langen ES, et al. Factors that predict prematurity and preeclampsia in pregnancies that are complicated by systemic lupus erythematosus. Am J Obstet Gynecol 2005;
5. Andrade R, Sanchez ML, Alarcón GS, et al. Adverse pregnancy outcomes in women with systemic lupus erythematosus from a multiethnic US cohort: LUMINA (LVI) [corrected]. Clin Exp Rheumatol 2008; 26:268.
6. Ross G, Sammaritano L, Nass R, Lockshin M. Effects of mothers' autoimmune disease during pregnancy on learning disabilities and hand preference in their children. Arch Pediatr Adolesc Med 2003; 157:397.
7. Izmirly PM, Costedoat-Chalumeau N, Pisoni CN, et al. Maternal use of hydroxychloroquine is associated with a reduced risk of recurrent anti-SSA/Ro-antibody-associated

cardiac manifestations of neonatal lupus. Circulation 2012; 126:76.
8. Lockshin MD, Sammaritano LR. Lupus pregnancy. Autoimmunity 2003; 36:33.
9. Andrade RM, McGwin G Jr, Alarcón GS, et al. Predictors of post-partum damage accrual in systemic lupus erythematosus: data from LUMINA, a multiethnic US cohort (XXXVIII). Rheumatology (Oxford) 2006; 45:1380.
10. Al-Herz A, Schulzer M, Esdaile JM. Survey of antimalarial use in lupus pregnancy and lactation. J Rheumatol 2002; 29:700.

65.25 Chapter 26 reference

1. Bar J, Ben-Rafael Z, Padoa A, et al. Prediction of pregnancy outcome in subgroups of women with renal disease. Clin Nephrol 2000; 53:437.
2. Imbasciati E, Gregorini G, Cabiddu G, et al. Pregnancy in CKD stages 3 to 5: fetal and maternal outcomes. Am J Kidney Dis 2007; 49:753.
3. Piccoli GB, Conijn A, Consiglio V, et al. Pregnancy in dialysis patients: is the evidence strong enough to lead us to change our counseling policy? Clin J Am Soc Nephrol 2010; 5:62.

65.26 Chapter 27 Reference

1. Royal College of Obstetricians and Gynaecologist. Green top guidelines. Anti-D immunoglobulin for Rh prophylaxis. RCOG, London, 2002.
2. Silva, M (Ed). Standards for blood banks and transfusion services. 24th ed. American Association of Blood Banks. Amercian Association of Blood Banks, Bethesda, MD, 2006

3. Kumpel BM. Analysis of factors affecting quantification of fetomaternal hemorrhage by flow cytometry. Transfusion 2000; 40:1376.
4. Lafferty J, Raby A, Keeney M, et al. Inaccurate doses of Rh immune globulin after Rh-incompatible fetomaternal hemorrhage-survey of laboratory practice. Arch Pathol Lab Med 2009; 133:1910.
5. Sandler SG, Gottschall JL. Postpartum Rh immunoprophylaxis. Obstet Gynecol 2012; 120:1428.
6. Wagner FF, Gassner C, Müller TH, et al. Molecular basis of weak D phenotypes. Blood 1999; 93:385.
7. Flegel WA. Molecular genetics and clinical applications for RH. Transfus Apher Sci 2011; 44:81

65.27 Chapter 28 Reference

1. Sabers A. Influences on seizure activity in pregnant women with epilepsy. Epilepsy Behav 2009; 15:230.
2. Morrow JI, Hunt SJ, Russell AJ, et al. Folic acid use and major congenital malformations in offspring of women with epilepsy: a prospective study from the UK Epilepsy and Pregnancy Register. J Neurol Neurosurg Psychiatry 2009; 80:506.
3. AAN guideline summary for clinicians. Management issues for women with epilepsy. www.aan.com/professionals/practice/pdfs/women_epilepsy.pdf (Accessed on March 7, 2005).
4. Meador KJ, Baker GA, Browning N, et al. Effects of breastfeeding in children of women taking antiepileptic drugs. Neurology 2010; 75:1954.

65.28 Chapter 29 Reference

1. Drenthen W, Pieper PG, Roos-Hesselink JW, et al. Outcome of pregnancy in women with congenital heart disease: a literature review. J Am Coll Cardiol 2007; 49:2303.
2. ACOG Committee on Practice Bulletins. ACOG Practice Bulletin No. 74. Antibiotic prophylaxis for gynecologic procedures. Obstet Gynecol 2006; 108:225.
3. Elkayam U, Bitar F. Valvular heart disease and pregnancy part I: native valves. J Am Coll Cardiol 2005; 46:223.
4. Siu SC, Sermer M, Colman JM, et al. Prospective multicenter study of pregnancy outcomes in women with heart disease. Circulation 2001; 104:515.

65.29 Reference Section II Instruction manual in Labour room

1. **Analgesia, anesthesia and pregnancy: a practical guide. Cambridge. 2007.**
2. **Antenatal Corticosteroids to Prevent Respiratory Distress Syndrome RCOG**
3. **Arad I. "Vacuum extraction at caesarean section neonatal outcome" J. Perinat. Med. 14 1986; 14: 137-140.**
4. **Best Practice in Labour and Delivery. Warren, Arulkumaran. Cambridge 2010.**
5. **'Birth after previous caesarean birth' Green top guideline No45 RCOG 2007**
6. **Caesarean section or vaginal delivery at 24 to 28 weeks gestation:**
   comparison of survival and neonatal and two-year morbidity. Kitchen W, Ford GW, Doyle LW, Rickards AL, Lissenden JV, Pepperell RH, Duke JE Obstet Gynecol 1985 Aug 66:2 149-157.

7. Changing prognosis for babies of less than 28 weeks gestation in the north of England between 1983 and 1994. Northern Neonatal Network. Tin W,Wariyar U, Hey E BMJ 1997 Jan 11;314 (7074): 107-11.
8. Child Fetal Neonatal Ed 1996 May 74:3 F214-8.
9. Fasubaa et al. Delivery of the impacted head of the fetus at caesarean section after prolonged obstructed labour: a randomised comparative study of two methods. Journal of Obstetrics and Gynaecology, 2002 Jul;22(4):375-378.
10. Flamm BL, Goings JR, Fuelberth N-J et al (1987) Oxytocin during labour after previous caesarean section: results of a multi-centre study. Obstetrics & Gynaecology 70: 709-12
11. Intrapartum Care for the MRCOG and beyond. RCOG Press.
12. Green–top Guideline No. 42
13. Green–top Guideline No. 56 January 2011
14. Journal of Perinatal Medicine, 2004, 32:465-469
15. K Clift & J Clift Uterine relaxation during caesarean section under regional anaesthesia: a survey of UK obstetric anaesthetists Int J or Obstet Anaesthesia.Oct 2008;17(4),374-375
16. Landesman, R, Graber, EA. Abdominovaginal delivery: modification of the cesarean section operation to facilitate delivery of the impacted head. Am J Obstet Gynecol 1984; 148:707.
17. Lydon-Rochelle M et al 2001: Risk of uterine rupture during labour among women with a prior Caesarean delivery New England Journal of Medicine 345(1):3-8
18. MacKenzie IZ, Bradley S, Embrey MP. (1984) Vaginal prostaglandins and labour induction for patients previously delivered by caesarean section. BJOG 91: 7-10

19. Management of Breech Presentation, RCOG Green-top guideline No 20B, December 2006
20. Management of genital Herpes in Pregnancy, RCOG Green-top guideline No. 30, September 2007
21. Meehan FP, Rafla NM, Burke G (1990) Regional epidural analgesia for labour following previous caesarean section. J.Obst.Gynaecol. 10: 312-6
22. Morton SC, Williams MS, Keeler EB et al Effect of epidural analgesia for labour on the caesarean delivery rate. Obstetr. Gynaecol. 1994 83(6): 1045-52
23. Nakano R. "Use of the vacuum extractor for delivery of the fetal head at caesarean section" Obstet. Gynecol.
24. NICE guidelines [CG190] Published date: December 2014
25. NICE guidelines [CG190] Published date: December 2014
26. NICE Guideline Caesarean Section Guideline 13 2004
27. NICE guideline Intrapartum Care 2007
28. Perinatal management at the lower limit of viability. JM Rennie Arch Dis
29. Prevention of Perinatal Group B Streptococcal Disease CDC, 2010
30. Saving Mothers Lives the seventh report of the Confidential Enquiries into Maternal Deaths in the United Kingdom. CEMACH London: December 2007
31. SOGC Guidelines for Vaginal Birth After Previous Caesarean Birth No 155 Feb 2005
32. Solomons E. "Delivery of the head by Malmstrom vacuum extractor during caesarean section" Obstet. Gynecol 1962; 19: 201.
33. Oxford specialist handbooks in anesthesia: Obstetric Anesthesia. Oxford. 2008.
34. Withholding or withdrawing Life Saving Treatment in Children – A Framework for Practice. Royal College of Paediatrics and Child Health, September 1997.

Printed in the United States
By Bookmasters